Essentials *of* CHEST RADIOLOGY

JOHN V. FORREST, M.D.
Professor of Radiology
Chief, Diagnostic Radiology
University of California, San Diego, School of Medicine
San Diego, California

DAVID S. FEIGIN, M.D.
Associate Professor of Radiology
University of California, San Diego, School of Medicine
Chief, Chest Radiology
Veterans Administration Medical Center
La Jolla, California

1982
W.B. SAUNDERS COMPANY
Philadelphia / London / Toronto / Mexico City / Rio de Janeiro / Sydney / Tokyo

W. B. Saunders Company: West Washington Square
                           Philadelphia, PA   19105

                           1 St. Anne's Road
                           Eastbourne, East Sussex BN21 3UN, England

                           1 Goldthorne Avenue
                           Toronto, Ontario M8Z 5T9, Canada

                           Apartado 26370—Cedro 512
                           Mexico 4, D.F., Mexico

                           Rua Coronel Cabrita, 8
                           Sao Cristovao Caixa Postal 21176
                           Rio de Janeiro, Brazil

                           9 Waltham Street
                           Artarmon, N.S.W. 2064, Australia

                           Ichibancho, Central Bldg., 22-1 Ichibancho
                           Chiyoda-Ku, Tokyo 102, Japan

Library of Congress Cataloging in Publication Data

Forrest, John V.

Essentials of chest radiology.

Bibliography: p.

Includes index.

1. Chest—Radiography.   2. Chest—Diseases—
   Diagnosis.   I. Feigin, David S.   II. Title.

RC941.F67   617'.5407572   82–47768
ISBN 0–7216–3818–X   AACR2

Essentials of Chest Radiology   ISBN   0-7216-3818-X

Last digit is the print number: 9   8   7   6   5   4   3   2   1

*To the medical students and
house officers at the University
of California, San Diego,
Washington University, the Johns
Hopkins Medical Institutions
and the Uniformed Services
University of the Health Sciences*

PREFACE

Our teachers and colleagues have always been very involved in training medical students and nonradiology house officers. We owe our interest and many of our techniques and abilities to them and would like to acknowledge their influence on our lives and skills. They include Harry Mellins, Dick Greenspan, Gerry Scanlon, Dave Rockoff, Jim Potchen, John Armstrong, Stu Sagel, Paul Friedman, Elliott Lasser, Martin Donner, Stan Siegelman, Fred Stitik, Lee Theros and John Madewell.

The enthusiasm and intelligence of students and house officers have been a constant source of pleasure and education during our careers in radiology. It is amazing how frequently the teacher becomes the one taught. A few of these individuals have even seen Roentgen's invisible light and become radiologists.

The Department of Radiology at the University of California, San Diego, has a generous policy of allowing sabbatical leave to all its members, even to those not involved in basic research. Without such time JVF would not have had the opportunity to put together the manual that formed the nucleus of this book. Our thanks to all our colleagues. Special gratitude to Paul Friedman for the extra work he did while John Forrest was writing and for helping edit the original manuscript.

Finally, we are indebted to a number of individuals who provided the technical, editorial, and secretarial assistance that made this book a pleasure to produce. The photography was beautifully executed by Yuji Oishi, M.D., of Denver, Colorado. The manuscript was flawlessly and efficiently typed in its many revisions by Barbara Messenger. Clare Latka provided significant secretarial and logistic assistance to us. Last, the production and editorial staff of W. B. Saunders Company, particularly Ms. Lisette Bralow, showed remarkable expertise in performing the myriad details involved in publication. Our deepest thanks to all these individuals.

JOHN V. FORREST, M.D.
DAVID S. FEIGIN, M.D.
San Diego, California

CONTENTS

INTRODUCTION

Findings on the roentgenogram may exhibit a pattern that allows a practical use of radiology in clinical problems. When it can be determined that a certain radiographic pattern is present, findings may be correlated with those on previous films and with other clinical information to allow a specific diagnosis. Occasionally the radiographic pattern alone allows the diagnosis, but more often it suggests a group of likely possibilities. Since the chest roentgenogram is often an early part of the workup, it may facilitate evaluation of the patient, eliminating unnecessary procedures.

Chapters 2 to 7 discuss the differential diagnosis of radiographic patterns or findings. Lillington and Jamplis have written an excellent book (see Bibliography) that uses this approach. Chapters 8 to 12 examine the diagnostic possibilities based on the location of an abnormality in the chest. The common diseases that affect the lungs are reviewed in Chapters 13 to 19. More elaborate discussions of these and less common diseases can be found in the textbook by Fraser and Paré (see Bibliography).

A key decision in the clinical-radiographic management of any patient is when to obtain a chest roentgenogram. More specifically, when not to get a film should be considered. Each clinician must manage the patient's clinical problem in his or her own way, but certain things should be checked.

1. Is a recent chest film already available?

2. Is the film being ordered because of some questionable "rule": as part of a physical examination, admission, preoperative workup or ICU routine?

3. Is the patient possibly pregnant? If the abdomen is well shielded, little or no radiation should reach the fetus. It is important to remember that a fetus is sensitive to radiation, more so earlier in pregnancy. Radiation causes teratogenesis and a significant increase in childhood leukemia.

CHAPTER 1

HINTS FOR READING CHEST ROENTGENOGRAMS

BASIC TECHNIQUE

Postero-anterior (PA).   This is the standard frontal chest roentgeno-gram with the patient facing the film cassette (Fig. 1–1). PA is the direction the x-rays travel going through the patient. This examination is taken with a tube film distance of six or more feet to reduce distortion caused by magnification of structures.

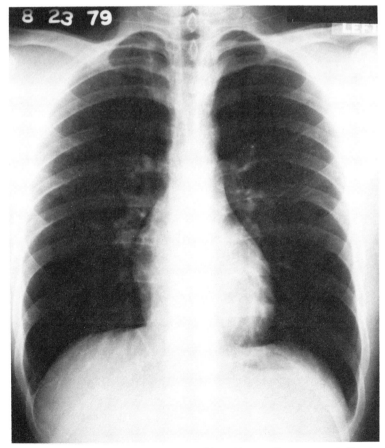

Figure 1–1. PA frontal chest film. This well-penetrated film in full inspiration shows the trachea clearly visible and the margins of the spine visible through the heart shadow. Both ribs and lung markings can be outlined.

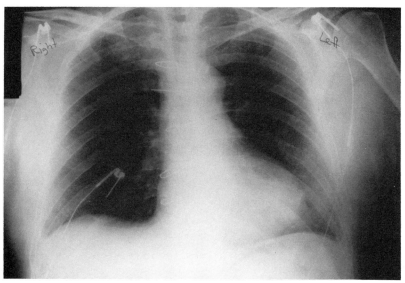

Figure 1–2. AP portable chest film. Despite compromises in technique because of portable equipment, the same basic features are visible as in the PA film (Fig. 1–1). As is typical, this sitting patient has not taken as deep a breath as he might if standing. Chest monitor leads and wire sutures in the sternum are seen.

Antero-posterior (AP). This is an alternate frontal film technique used in patients who are difficult to position for a PA view. This projection (Fig. 1–2) causes some increase in apparent cardiac size, especially if the tube–film distance is short. This examination is often made with portable equipment, which also has the problems of less power and inconsistent power. AP chest films are often semilordotic (patient leaning back with clavicles higher than usual relative to the ribs), and poor contact between patient and film increases blurring of structures.

Lateral. This projection (Fig. 1–3) is a right angle view complementary to the PA or AP film. Several recent studies have suggested a limited value for this widely used view, particularly if a kVp (see Glossary if definition needed) of 120 or more is used for the frontal radiograph. This view does allow confirmation of the presence and location of an abnormality, especially in or near the hilum (see Chapter 9). It also provides the best view of the posterior lung bases and the retrosternal area.

Overpenetrated PA or AP. Use of greater mAs (see Glossary) allows more x-rays to pass through the patient and strike the film (Fig. 1–4). Lung detail is poor, but the spine and mediastinum are well seen.

Obliques. Another way of confirming the presence, location and shape of an abnormality, these views (Figs. 1–5 and 1–6) are used when the PA and lateral views do not both show the finding. Mediastinal and hilar contour can be examined to advantage with oblique views. To orient yourself to oblique views, follow the trachea to the carina and note how the hilar structures surround the main stem bronchi. On the LAO (left anterior oblique) view (Fig. 1–5) the trachea moves to the patient's right of the spine, and on the RAO (right anterior oblique) view (Fig. 1–6) the trachea swings to the patient's left of the spine. The LAO view is exactly the same as the RPO (right posterior oblique) view except for minimal

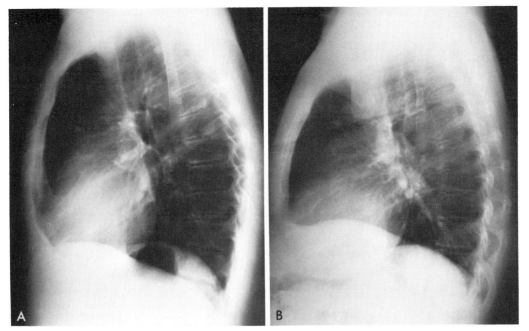

Figure 1–3. Standard lateral chest view. *A,* Evidence that this patient is properly positioned includes the observations that the turning points of the ribs posterior to the spine overlap each other and that the two posterior costophrenic angles are aligned vertically. *B,* For comparison, another lateral film of this patient shows poor positioning.

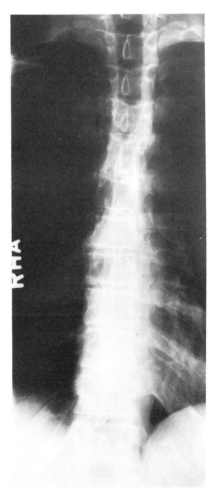

Figure 1–4. Overpenetrated frontal chest film. This film, obtained to view the thoracic spine, uses technique that overexposes the heart, hila and lung fields. Because it is directly over the spine, the trachea is more visible than with standard technique.

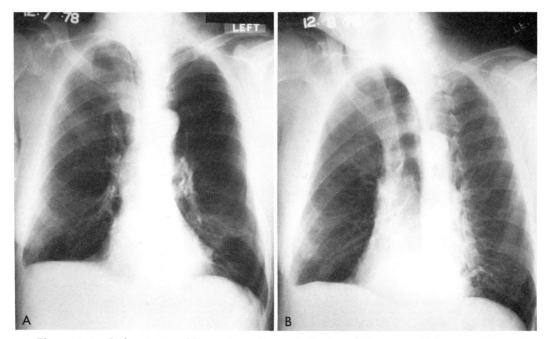

Figure 1–5. Left anterior oblique chest films. *A*, Shallow oblique. *B*, 45-degree oblique. For both films, the patient has turned towards his right so that the anterior structures (such as medial clavicles and trachea) are to the right of his posterior structures (spine). To orient yourself, follow the trachea to the carina; the hila surround each main bronchus.

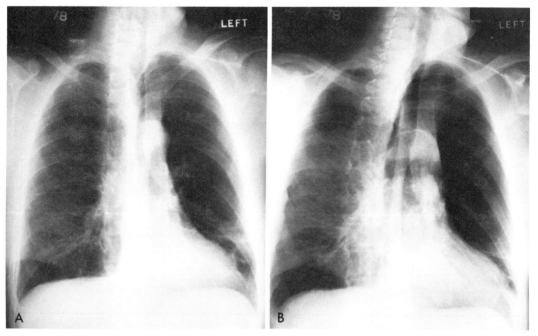

Figure 1–6. Right anterior oblique chest films. *A*, Shallow. *B*, Slightly more steep. Here the trachea and medial clavicles are to the patient's left of the posterior midline spine. Again, use the trachea and main bronchi for orientation.

changes in magnification and distortion. Shallow obliques (Figs. 1–5*A* and 1–6*A*) are best for viewing lung fields and hilar structures, while 45 degree obliques show the heart and great vessels somewhat better.

Lateral Decubitus. This frontal film is taken with the patient lying on one side (Fig. 1–7). Documentation and quantitation of free pleural effusion are possible. Occasionally this is the best technique to use to demonstrate a pneumothorax. The lung hidden behind a pleural effusion may be seen with this projection. It is usually necessary to obtain both lateral decubitus views when a patient may have a significant pleural effusion. The decubitus view with the abnormal side up is the best one for viewing the lung and is especially important for seeing if a pulmonary infiltrate is present in addition to the effusion.

Apical Lordotic. This is an AP view with the patient arching his back and resting his shoulders against the film holder (Fig. 1–8). By this maneuver the clavicle and anterior first rib are projected above the lung fields, allowing visualization of subtle lesions obscured on the PA view. The extreme lung apex is not evaluated by this projection. Use of standard films with a kVp of 120 or more eliminates most of the need for this projection, since higher kV x-rays penetrate bone to show underlying abnormalities.

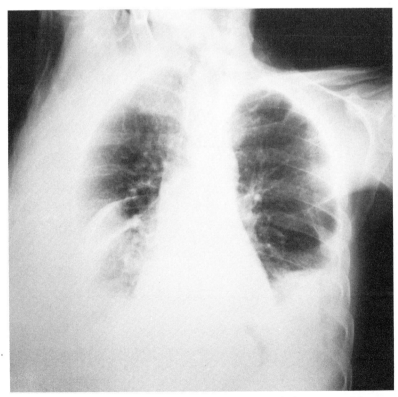

Figure 1–7. Right lateral decubitus view. With this patient lying on his right side, a large pleural effusion is seen that was not evident on frontal and lateral views (see Fig. 12–4). Fluid is thickening the lateral portion of the fissures in the right lung.

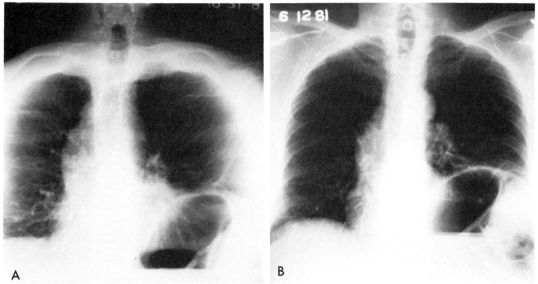

Figure 1–8. *A,* Apical lordotic chest view. *B,* Standard PA view of same patient. Note the change in position of clavicles and anterior first ribs.

Fluoroscopy. Movement of intrathoracic structures can be best appreciated with this technique. Cardiovascular abnormalities, particularly calcifications, and diaphragmatic motion are well evaluated.

Tomography (Laminography). Synchronous movement of the film holder and the x-ray tube blurs all but one plane of the structure filmed (Fig. 1–9). The level of this plane is measured in centimeters from the table top. Current uses include the following:

1. Evaluation for a hilar mass (often 55 degree posterior oblique is the best projection).
2. Determination of the exact location of an abnormality (used before bronchoscopy, needle aspiration, or surgery).
3. Examination for small nodules in metastatic disease.
4. Examination for calcification or cavitation (usually can be done more simply with oblique views or fluoroscopy).
5. Evaluation for mediastinal mass (CT better).
6. Documentation of the characteristic shape and course of certain parenchymal lesions (bronchocele, arteriovenous malformation, varix, anomalous vein).

BAD TECHNIQUE

Bad technique often leads to misreadings of chest films. Underexposure will cause abnormalities to hide next to or behind bony or mediastinal shadows. Overexposure may cause small or poorly defined abnormalities to be difficult to see, or even to disappear. A properly penetrated chest film should allow visualization of small pulmonary vessels almost to the edge of the lungs (Fig. 1–1). Pulmonary blood vessels and disc spaces of the thoracic spine should be barely visible through the cardiac shadow.

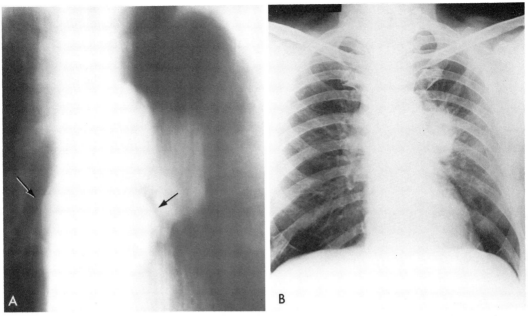

Figure 1–9. *A*, Frontal tomogram. Arrows point to bronchi. *B*, Standard frontal view of same patient. The tomogram, focused at the plane just posterior to the carina, shows the branching of the normal right bronchus and inferior displacement of the left bronchus by a large mass (squamous carcinoma) just anterolateral to the descending aorta.

A correctly centered PA or AP film will have the medial clavicles approximately the same distance from the midline (the spinous processes) (Figs. 1–5*A* and 1–6*A* compared with Fig. 1–1). Rotation may hide abnormalities or cause a normal mediastinal contour to be misjudged as abnormal.

Maximum inspiration during exposure of the radiograph is necessary to see the lung fields adequately, judge hilar and vascular shadows, and evaluate the mediastinal contour, particularly heart size. If the <u>anterior</u> end of the <u>right sixth rib</u> is visible above the right hemidiaphragm on the PA film, inspiration is adequate. *or 10th Post. Rib*

Another useful index of adequate inspiration is a heart shadow that is completely visible above the left hemidiaphragm. If the heart appears to be "hiding" behind the diaphragm, the inspiration is probably inadequate. Patient lack of cooperation, pain, intra-abdominal disease, and obesity are common causes of inadequate inspiration.

ARTIFACTS

Film artifact is a common problem. Foreign bodies outside the patient and abnormal densities due to film handling or processing may cause artifacts (Fig. 1–10). It is important, however, to remember that an unusual density may be a foreign body inside the patient that may be of great clinical importance. Frequently, ingested or inhaled objects, bullets and shrapnel are ignored because they are mistaken for artifacts.

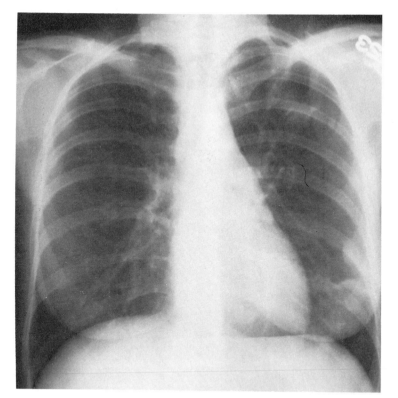

Figure 1–10. Frontal chest film with artifacts. Several densities, caused by clothing, are seen over the lateral portion of the left lung field, thus resembling pulmonary infiltrates. In this case, the densities are very difficult to identify as artifacts, as they do not continue laterally beyond the lung field.

Figure 1–11. Cutaneous mass projecting over lung. This pedunculated skin polyp is attached only medially to the skin, accounting for the sharp borders in all other directions.

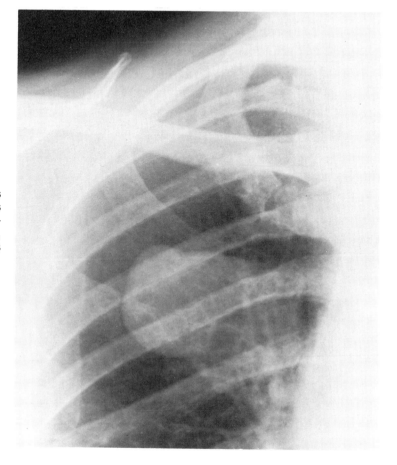

SKIN LESIONS

A wide variety of soft tissue and skin structures and abnormalities may produce densities on the chest radiograph. A protuberant density that is well marginated by external air can produce an apparent lung nodule or mass. Sometimes the sharp margin of this density is a clue to its true location (Fig. 1–11). A common example of this problem is the normal nipple, which may be seen unilaterally or bilaterally. Films taken with nipple markers may be necessary to determine if a density is the nipple. Often inspection of the patient will confirm or reveal the skin or soft tissue cause of an enigmatic shadow.

Breasts also frequently cause confusing findings on the chest roentgenogram. Surgical removal, congenital or acquired aplasia or hypoplasia can create an asymmetrical appearance that is easily mistaken for lung disease (Fig. 1–12). Small dense breasts also create problems in interpretation. These are often seen in teenage girls or in men with gynecomastia. The problem is compounded when significant asymmetry of the breasts is present. Particularly when pressed against the film-holding device in the PA projection, small dense breasts mimic lung consolidation. Familiarity with this problem, its typical location, correlation with the lateral film, and examination of the patient are all helpful in avoiding a misdiagnosis.

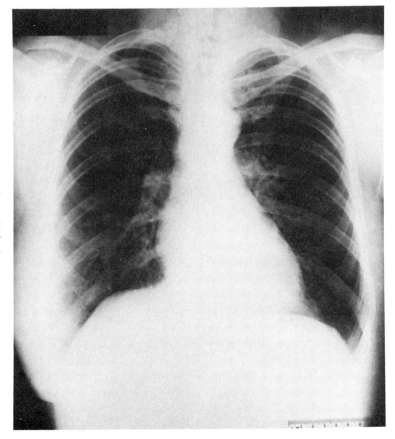

Figure 1–12. Frontal film with left mastectomy. Note how the asymmetry of soft tissues creates the impression of excessive density in the lateral portion of the right lower lung field that could be mistaken for a pneumonia or pleural thickening.

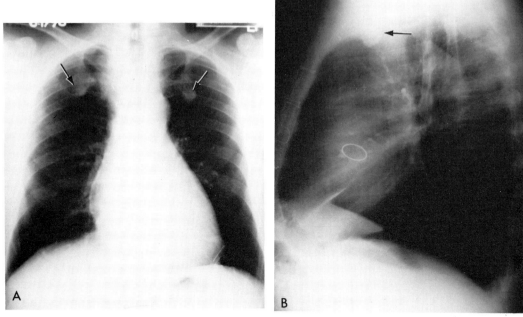

Figure 1–13. Prominent first costochondral junctions. *A,* Frontal view. *B,* Lateral view. Although asymmetry is common, there is usually some enlargement of the contralateral costochondral junction whenever one junction is so obvious that it resembles a mass.

RIBS

Since ribs overlie the lungs, variations and abnormalities in these bones are frequently misinterpreted as pulmonary abnormalities. Normal variations such as bifid rib, fused ribs or hypoplastic ribs can be a problem. Healing and healed rib fractures are commonly mistaken for pulmonary nodules. Often, appropriately obliqued films are necessary to resolve this difficulty. The costochondral junction and costochondral calcification also are frequently mistaken for abnormal lung densities. This is particularly true of the first costochondral junction, which characteristically is hyperplastic, irregular and sometimes asymmetric (Fig. 1–13). Many patients have received elaborate workups for cancer, tuberculosis and other problems because of a prominent first costochondral junction. Any other form of local rib abnormality can be mistaken for a lung lesion by the unwary (Fig. 1–14).

Occasionally, diffuse rib disease, particularly blastic metastases, is mistaken for diffuse lung disease. Diffuse, homogeneous increase in bony density may accentuate underlying pulmonary vascular and interstitial markings, leading to this error.

LUNG BASES

It should always be remembered that a significant portion of the pulmonary parenchyma lies below the levels of the most superior portions of the hemidiaphragms. This is obvious when one notes the shape of the hemidiaphragms on the lateral view (Fig. 1–3). The effect is markedly

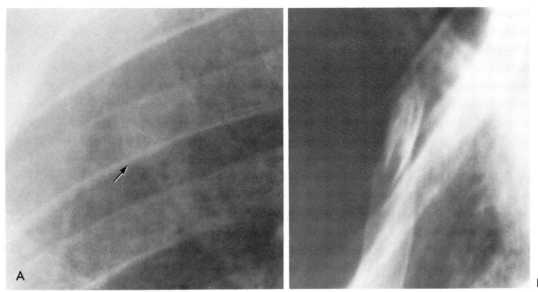

Figure 1–14. Rib fracture resembling lung mass. *A*, Mass (arrow) appears present in right upper lobe of a PA chest film. *B*, Oblique view taken at fluoroscopy shows displaced rib fracture. Overlap of rib fragments caused the shadow on the PA view.

enhanced if the patient is positioned in lordosis (as in Fig. 1–8*A*). Overpenetrated views of the lower lung fields may be very helpful in evaluating these areas if a film of the abdomen is not already available.

THE WRONG PATIENT

Misdiagnosis and confusion are frequently caused by unlabeled or mislabeled films. Films on one patient may end up in another patient's jacket. Any very rapid change or unexpected finding should raise the possibility that the films are not of the correct patient. In instances in which the films are improperly labeled, this determination may be difficult, but careful comparison of known stable structures on serial films is often conclusive. Nodal and cartilage calcification rarely change significantly. Bony contours and variations are also reliable standards of comparison.

A SYSTEMATIC APPROACH

Radiologists vary in their method of reading chest radiographs. Some study the whole film using a recognition pattern, while others use a mental check list to review systematically all areas and information. Both methods seem effective for experienced individuals.

Beginners or those who do not regularly look at chest radiographs are better off with a systematic approach to avoid omission. Any routine is acceptable. For example, the following may be used:

1. Check film quality.
2. Look at the *neck* for calcification, soft tissue asymmetry, airway abnormalities.

3. Follow the *trachea and bronchi* as far as they can be seen.
4. Examine the *shoulders, clavicles, scapulae, sternum, spine* and *ribs* for symmetry, deformity, fracture, dislocation and lytic or blastic areas.
5. Examine the *soft tissues*, including the breasts, for symmetry, calcification, masses and irregularity.
6. Check the *area beneath the diaphragm* for free or loculated air, abnormality of soft tissue, hollow organs and calcification.
7. Look at *diaphragmatic* position, contour and possible calcification.
8. Trace out the normal *pleural surfaces*, searching for evidence of free or loculated effusion, adhesions and calcification. Note the position and appearance of major, minor and accessory *fissures.*
9. Examine the *mediastinal and hilar contour* for position and density.
10. Search the *lung fields* systematically. Pay particular attention to the apices and the areas around the hila and superior mediastinum, since small lesions are often partially hidden by overlying bones and blood vessels in these areas. Subtle air bronchograms or examples of the silhouette sign are often the best clues to a small parenchymal consolidation.

COMPARISON WITH OTHER RADIOGRAPHS

The chronology of a finding on the chest radiograph is often critical for diagnosis and management. Unless careful comparison with both recent and remote previous radiographs is regularly made, major error will occur. The inconvenience of tracking down previous studies in your own institution or from other sources often causes this comparison to be omitted. Of all the major causes of patient mismanagement from radiologic data, this is one of the most common. Remember that portions of the chest are frequently included on films of other structures and such films can be used for comparison.

Variation in film technique and processing may cause differences on the films that are mistakenly called worsening or improvement. This is particularly true on portable examinations. A good general rule is not to alter patient management on the basis of questionable radiographic change.

CHAPTER 2

CONSOLIDATION

Consolidation usually indicates an alveolar filling process, since it is due to the accumulation of abnormal material in the air spaces. Characteristics of consolidation (Fig. 2–1) include the following:

1. confluence within areas of involvement
2. indistinct margins, unless the density ends at a peripheral pleural surface or fissure
3. frequent air bronchograms
4. obliteration of vascular shadows
5. the silhouette sign

This form of abnormal density is often patchy or nonhomogeneous as "alveolar nodules" (Fig. 2–2). When it is homogeneous and dense, it may mimic a mass (Fig. 2–3). If it is faint and patchy, it may be indistinguishable from a primary interstitial disease process.

The term consolidation is preferable to "alveolar" because severe, diffuse interstitial disease can mimic the roentgenographic findings of alveolar filling and appear as consolidation (Fig. 2–4). This occurs because confluent thickening of the interstitium can squeeze the air out of intervening alveoli so that no air remains in that area of the lung.

Consolidation may also result from mixed alveolar filling and interstitial disease (Fig. 2–2). When both alveolar filling and interstitial thickening occur in the same area of lung at the same time, the alveolar filling obscures the linear reticulations of interstitial thickening by depriving the lung of the air lucencies between the thickened elements of the interstitium. For this reason, alveolar filling (or collapse) "masks" interstitial disease.

Causes of consolidation include:

A. Local
   1. Lobar or segmental: infection, particularly pneumococcal pneumonia (Figs. 2–3, 2–5), infarction
   2. Patchy: infection, aspiration, contusion, allergic response, edema, radiation damage (Fig. 2–6), neoplasm, vasculitis
   3. Mass-like: infarction, infection, hematoma, neoplasm (Fig. 2–7), radiation damage
B. Diffuse: edema, aspiration, infection, hemorrhage (Fig. 2–2), allergic reaction, adult respiratory distress syndrome (many causes), neoplasm (Fig. 2–7), alveolar proteinosis (Fig. 2–1)

It is worth remembering that the consolidative pattern is most often caused by hemorrhage, exudate or edema—*"blood, pus or water."* This catch phrase is generally the most useful place from which to begin your differential diagnosis of consolidation. If those causes are excluded, try *"protein or cells."*

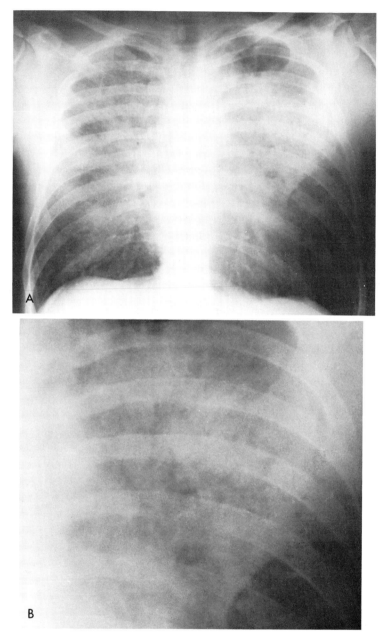

Figure 2–1. Diffuse consolidation of alveolar proteinosis. This moderately rare disease fills alveolar spaces but leaves the interstitium completely normal. All the characteristics of consolidation are visible. The air bronchogram is best seen in the left upper lung field on the closeup (*B*) (AFIP negative #73–11972).

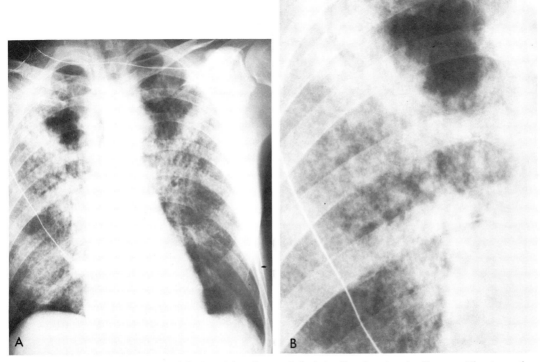

Figure 2–2. Patchy consolidation (alveolar nodules) in Goodpasture's disease. The irregular nodules of hemorrhage, especially evident in the closeup of the right upper lung field (*B*), fill all the criteria of consolidation. On biopsy, interstitial thickening was found as well as alveolar filling, but the interstitial disease was largely "masked" by the patchy alveolar consolidation. A reticular interstitial pattern (see Chapter 4) is probably present in the periphery and in the right lower lung field, where less consolidation is present.

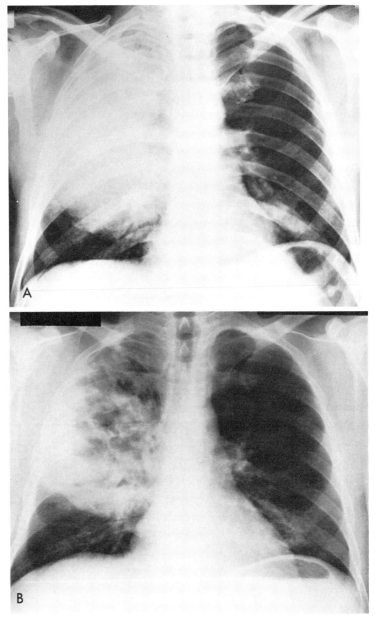

Figure 2–3. Pneumococcal pneumonia, right upper lobe. *A,* Initial film shows complete consolidation of right upper lobe, with massive expansion forcing the fissures downward. *B,* Film five days later with partial clearing shows air bronchograms, areas of cleared alveoli appearing as cysts and minimal decrease in hyperexpansion of the right upper lobe. Areas of cleared lung, as here, may be indistinguishable from cavities representing pulmonary necrosis.

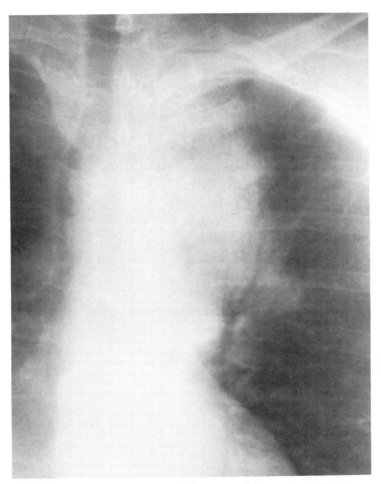

Figure 2–4. Lymphoma, left upper lobe and mediastinum. When pulmonary lymphoma infiltrates the lung, the interstitium is so massively thickened that consolidation, with an air bronchogram, may result (AFIP negative #73–2069).

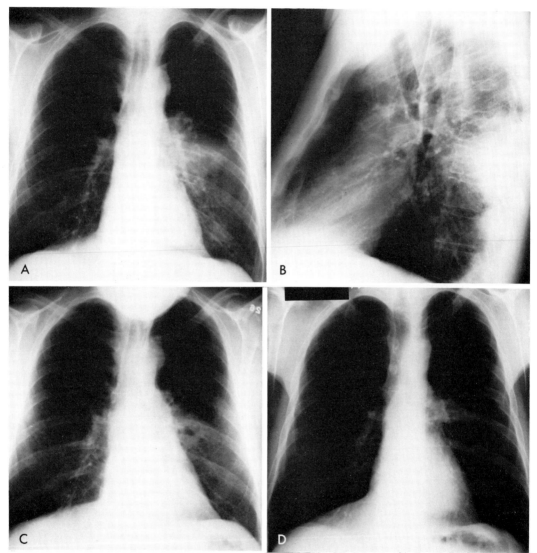

Figure 2–5. Segmental pneumonia. *A* and *B*, Frontal and lateral initial films show consolidation in superior segment of left lower lobe. Typical consolidation is seen without an air bronchogram, suggesting some bronchial obstruction. *C*, Followup film six days later shows cystic cavitation of the pneumonia. *D*, Another film, two weeks later, shows scarring lateral to the left hilum and minimal distortion of the hilum, both because of scarring from this destructive pneumonia.

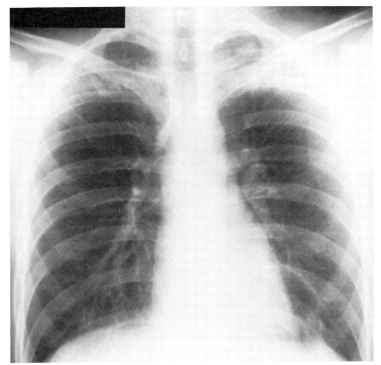

Figure 2–6. Radiation pneumonitis, both apices. This patient with Hodgkin's disease had radiation therapy in which the portals included the apices bilaterally. Hazy consolidation is visible in both upper lung fields and is indistinguishable from inflammation from other causes such as infection, including active tuberculosis.

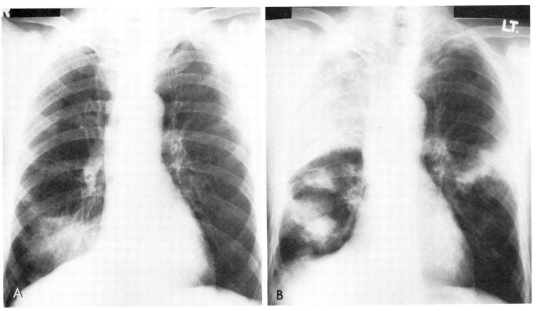

Figure 2–7. Alveolar cell carcinoma, right lower lobe, becoming diffuse. This unusual form of bronchogenic carcinoma often begins as a localized consolidation (*A*). It may subsequently spread via the bronchi to involve both lungs (*B*); the right upper lobe is completely consolidated, and there are patchy consolidations elsewhere.

CHAPTER 3

ATELECTASIS

Atelectasis is also called collapse or volume loss. An entire lung, a lobe, a segment or a subsegment may collapse, often showing characteristic radiographic findings, including abnormal lines or increased density in the involved part of the lung. When collapse of an entire lung is present, there is displacement of the mediastinum and diaphragm towards the involved lung unless either or both of these structures are fixed in position (Fig. 3–1).

With lobar atelectasis the mediastinal and diaphragmatic shift is less marked, but characteristic displacement of fissures and the hilum is seen (Fig. 3–2). Careful observation will frequently show increased lucency of the remaining overexpanded lung on the involved side, with spreading of the vasculature.

Causes of atelectasis include:

A. Total lung, lobar or segmental atelectasis: neoplasm (Figs. 3–2, 3–3, 3–4), foreign body (Fig. 3–1), misplaced endotracheal tube, secretions, mucous plugs, extrinsically compressing lymph nodes (Fig. 3–5), scarring, blood clots, broncholiths

B. Subsegmental (discoid, platelike): secretions, splinting for any reason, particularly chest or abdominal pain, pulmonary embolism

When the lung fields are asymmetric, a frequent problem is the inability to decide whether the underexpanded lung is abnormal or whether the contralateral overexpanded lung is abnormal (emphysematous). The decision can most easily be made by obtaining a film in full expiration. The mediastinum will swing towards the normal lung regardless of the position of the mediastinum on the inspiratory film. Such a swing is explained by the fact that the normal lung dispels the most air during expiration regardless of which lung is abnormally ventilated.

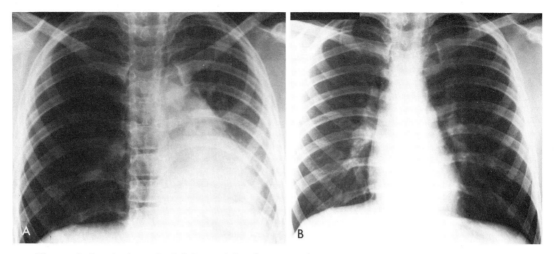

Figure 3–1. Atelectasis, left lower lobe, because of foreign body. *A,* Initial film shows marked deviation of mediastinum towards the left, increased density in left lower lung field and elevation of left hemidiaphragm. *B,* Film following bronchoscopic removal of foreign body shows return to full ventilation of left lower lobe.

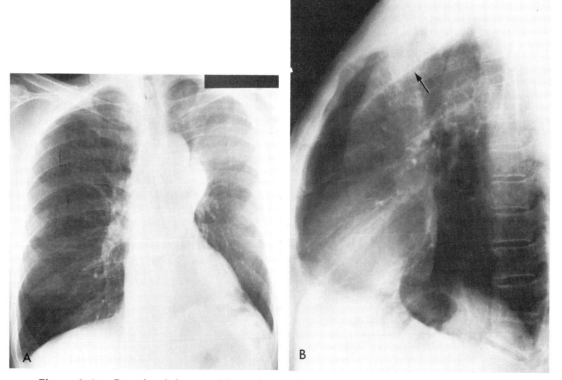

Figure 3–2. Complete left upper lobe atelectasis by bronchogenic carcinoma. Mediastinal shift, elevated left hemidiaphragm, distortion of left hilum with increased density and overall left lung volume loss are evident on frontal film (*A*). Lateral film (*B*) shows marked displacement of major fissure anterior and superior (arrow), a highly characteristic finding for left upper lobe atelectasis.

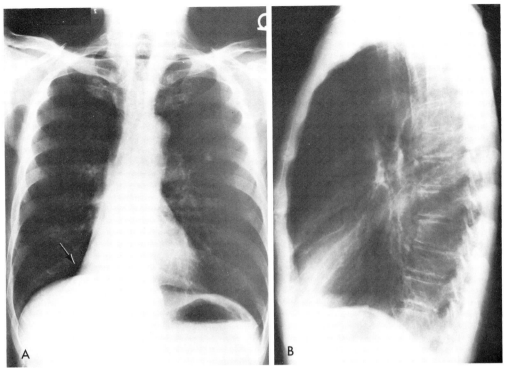

Figure 3–3. Complete right lower lobe atelectasis by bronchogenic carcinoma. On the frontal view (A) the major fissure is visible behind the heart, extending behind the right hemidiaphragm as well (arrow). Overall right volume loss is more subtle than in Figures 3–1 and 3–2. Lateral film (B) shows no significant abnormality other than poor visualization of the right hemidiaphragm. Atelectasis is often evident on one view and inapparent on the opposite (90 degrees different) view.

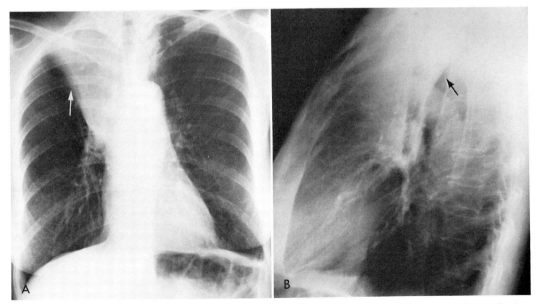

Figure 3–4. Partial right upper lobe atelectasis by bronchogenic carcinoma. A, Frontal view shows "S sign of Golden," which is superior displacement of minor fissure (arrow) with downward convexity near the hilum because of the mass itself. B, Anterior and superior displacement of major fissure on the lateral view (arrow) is less severe than in complete atelectasis, as in Figure 3–2.

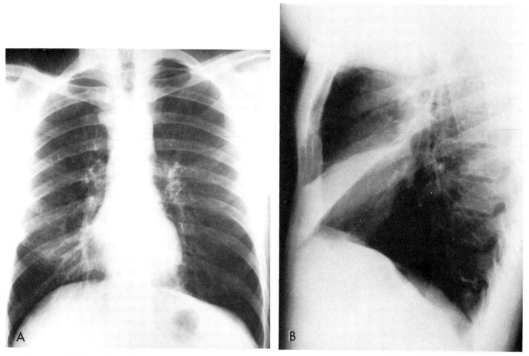

Figure 3–5. Partial right middle lobe atelectasis ("middle lobe syndrome"), probably lymph node compression. *A,* Frontal film shows hazy right heart border but no other abnormality. *B,* Lateral view shows increased density and sharp definition of middle lobe, with downward displacement of minor fissure and upward displacement of major fissure.

CHAPTER 4

INTERSTITIAL DISEASE

Abnormal thickening of lung interstitium may be manifest as many different radiographic patterns. The most typical signs of interstitial lung disease are the reticular pattern and septal (Kerley) lines (Figs. 4–1 and 4–2). Fine branching lines constitute a reticular pattern. When these lines are thicker and more confluent and form cystic spaces, the term "honeycomb" is often used (Fig. 4–3).

Kerley B lines are dilated interlobular septa that abut the pleura and extend for several millimeters (up to about 2 cm.) medially (Fig. 4–2). They cannot be followed into the hila, as can vessels and bronchi. Kerley B lines are best seen at the lung bases and are often the only sign of interstitial thickening when such thickening is mild and diffuse. Kerley A lines (Fig. 4–4) are also dilated interlobular septa, but these extend from the hilum to the periphery, usually in the upper lung fields. They are difficult to differentiate from vessels and are never seen without Kerley B lines or reticulations. "Kerley C lines" is simply another term for reticulations.

Radiographic patterns of interstitial disease without reticulations or septal lines are often not clearly definable as a primary interstitial process. Amorphous scattered densities, small irregular shadows and small nodules all fall into this category. Mixtures of these patterns are common. Severe interstitial thickening may collapse the surrounding air spaces and cause large or poorly marginated shadows with air bronchograms, which is typical of alveolar involvement (see Chapter 2).

Interstitial lung disease is typically diffuse, but any of its forms may be asymmetric or local. Occasionally, distribution helps in differential diagnosis. For example, chronic basilar disease is often caused by asbestosis (Fig. 4–5), scleroderma or rheumatoid disease. Upper lobe reticulonodular patterns are frequently caused by pneumoconiosis and eosinophilic granuloma. Interstitial diseases almost never have a distribution in specific bronchopulmonary segments, as seen in many consolidative diseases, such as pneumonia or atelectasis.

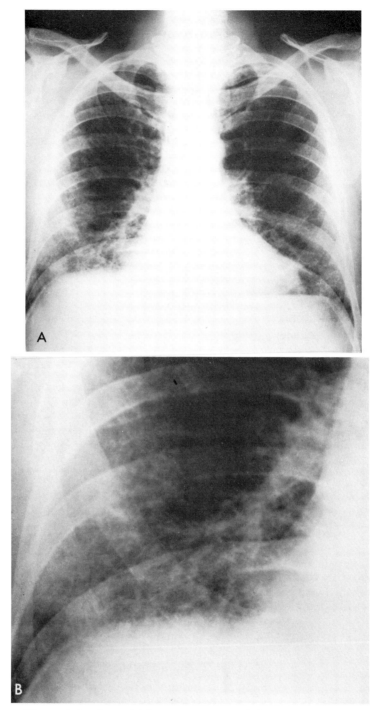

Figure 4–1. Interstitial pneumonia, probably allergic ("allergic alveolitis"). The frontal film (A) and closeup of right lower lung field (B) show bilateral lower lobe reticulations—lines running in every direction, including directions not possible by the normal bronchi and vessels. The upper lung fields are more normal, and there is minimal overall volume loss in the lungs.

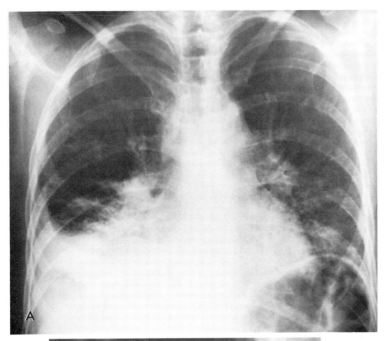

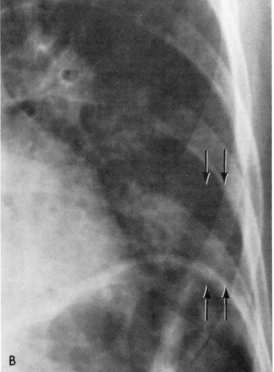

Figure 4–2. Interstitial pattern caused by lymphangitic spread of carcinoma (primary unknown). Frontal film (*A*) and closeup of left lower lung field (*B*) show reticulations that are far more irregular than those in Figure 4–1. Septal lines (Kerley B lines) are evident near the left costophrenic angle (between arrows) as a series of horizontal lines. The film also shows mediastinal widening and a large right pleural effusion.

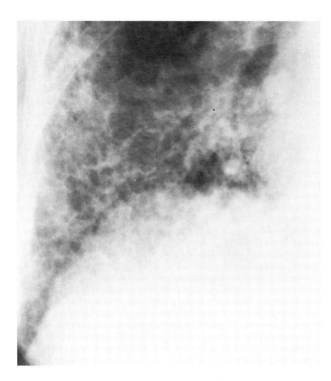

Figure 4–3. "Honeycomb lung." Irregular reticulations are forming irregular cystic spaces, especially in the periphery of the right lower lobe of this lung. If most of the lung were involved, the term "end stage lung" could be used.

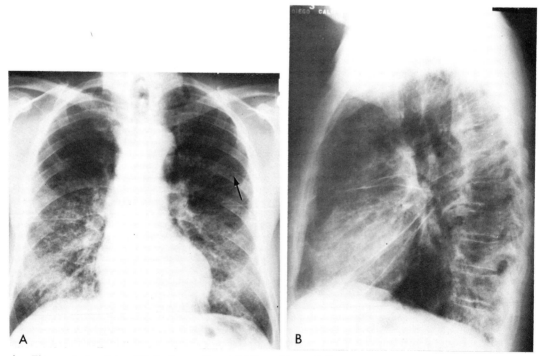

Figure 4–4. Interstitial edema. Frontal (*A*) and lateral (*B*) views show diffuse lower lung field reticulations, thickened fissures, septal lines, including Kerley A lines (arrow), and minimal dilatation of upper lobe vessels. In this case, there are no distinctive findings to distinguish edema from other causes of the interstitial pattern.

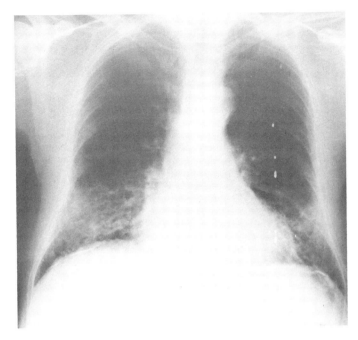

Figure 4–5. Asbestosis. Bilateral lower lobe reticulations are evident. Pathognomonic for asbestosis are the linear calcifications of both hemidiaphragms. Without these calcifications, this film could depict nearly any lower lobe interstitial disease.

ACUTE

The most common cause of acute interstitial thickening is edema (Fig. 4–4). Congestive heart failure is the usual reason, but any condition resulting in leakage of fluid from the vascular bed will cause acute edema.

Infections are another frequent cause of acute interstitial disease. Most often these are viral or mycoplasmal. Acute interstitial disease may also be caused by drug reaction or allergy (Fig. 4–1).

Lymphangitic spread of carcinoma (Fig. 4–2) is an important cause of interstitial disease, which appears superficially to resemble interstitial edema. It is vital to remember that diffuse interstitial disease has many other causes besides edema.

CHRONIC

Fibrosis is by far the most common of the chronic causes of the interstitial pattern (Fig. 4–3). In many instances no specific cause can be found. Any disease that diffusely damages the lung may eventually lead to fibrosis ("end stage" or true "honeycomb" lung).

Pathologists use the term "honeycomb" to refer only to architecturally distorted lung that is the product of scarring following severe alveolar wall damage. The term should really be reserved for such "end stage lung" and not used for every pattern of reticulations that one sees roentgenographically. In general, true "honeycomb lung" can be recognized by irregular interstitial thickening and irregular cystic spaces that extend far into the periphery of the lung (Fig. 4–3).

Other forms of a chronic interstitial pattern include residua of sarcoidosis, neoplasm, eosinophilic granuloma, the pneumoconioses, collagen vascular disease, particularly rheumatoid disease and scleroderma, hemosiderosis, bronchiectasis and bronchiolitis obliterans.

Unless a typical reticular or honeycomb pattern is seen, labeling diffuse lung disease "interstitial" is risky. It is more appropriate to term these other patterns "indeterminate," so that diffuse alveolar processes are not excluded. For example, early pulmonary alveolar proteinosis may present radiographically with diffuse, small amorphous shadows similar to an interstitial pattern.

Significant abnormality of the pulmonary interstitium may be present without radiographic findings. Evaluation of the arterial blood gases will often allow such a disease process to be suspected when the radiograph is not helpful, as a diffusion abnormality is a more sensitive index than visible interstitial infiltration in mild interstitial disease.

CHAPTER 5

NODULES AND MASSES

Solid densities in the lung have a wide variety of causes. Occasionally the radiographic findings suggest a particular entity, but usually this is not so. Unless a lesion has detectable calcification or is stable in size over at least two years, pathologic or microbiologic diagnosis is usually necessary, as the mass may be malignant.

Any calcification is evidence against malignancy, although rarely calcification will be present adjacent to a neoplasm. A central ("bull's eye") calcification or symmetrical lamellar calcification strongly suggests the diagnosis of a granuloma (Fig. 5–1). Whirls and swirls of calcification resembling the form of popcorn ("popcorn calcifications") are typical of some hamartomas.

Common causes of diffuse tiny nodules include granulomatous infection (often a miliary pattern), sarcoidosis, neoplasm, eosinophilic granuloma and silicosis (Fig. 5–2).

Multiple scattered nodules (0.5–3.0 cm. in diameter) (Fig. 5–3) may be caused by neoplasm (especially metastases), sarcoidosis, granulomatous infection, infarctions, silicosis, rheumatoid disease, vasculitis, septic emboli and arteriovenous malformations. In general, small, sharp, well-defined and evenly distributed nodules have originated in the interstitium of the lung and are caused by hematogenous metastatic disease or granulomatous diseases (infectious or noninfectious). Large, ill-defined, fluffy and unevenly distributed nodules generally have the same causes as alveolar consolidations (see Chapter 2). Areas of true consolidation with air bronchograms are often seen when alveolar nodules are present roentgenographically.

Any of the causes of nodular lesions listed above may also present as a solitary nodule or mass. Most solitary nodules are due to neoplasm, granuloma, hamartoma, abscess or infarction (Fig. 5–4). Less common causes are pneumonia, sequestration, varix and arteriovenous malformation. Chest wall lesions (nipple, mole, wen, lipoma, healed rib fracture) and pleural and artifactual shadows often mimic lung nodules (see Chapter 1). If the PA and lateral films do not localize the nodule to the lung parenchyma, correlation with physical examination or appropriate oblique views is necessary to confirm its location. When in doubt about the identity of any nodule or mass, the possibility of carcinoma must always be excluded by further investigation, which is often as simple as comparison of current films with old films.

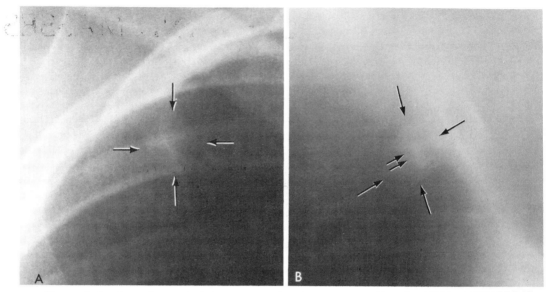

Figure 5–1. Granuloma, probably histoplasmosis, right upper lobe. *A,* Closeup of frontal view shows poorly defined nodule near periphery of lung, partially obscured by posterior and anterior ribs. *B,* Tomogram in steep oblique position shows calcification (double arrow) in center of mass. The tomogram obviates further workup for malignancy.

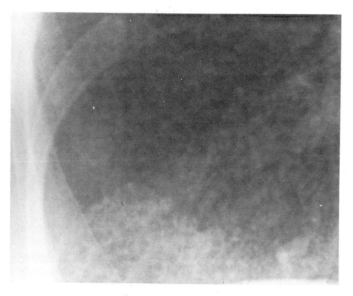

Figure 5–2. Miliary nodules of miliary tuberculosis. Multiple tiny, uniform nodules are easily seen in this closeup view of the right lower lung field. Nodules with this appearance nearly always represent nodular thickening of the pulmonary interstitium.

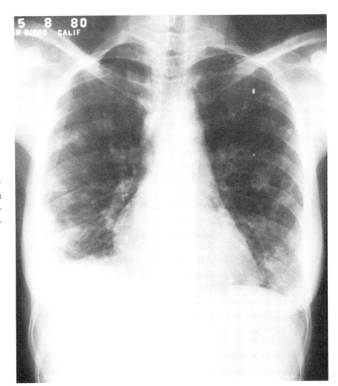

Figure 5–3. Septic emboli as multiple cavitated nodules. The nodules vary in size and shape and are unevenly distributed. A right pleural effusion is also evident.

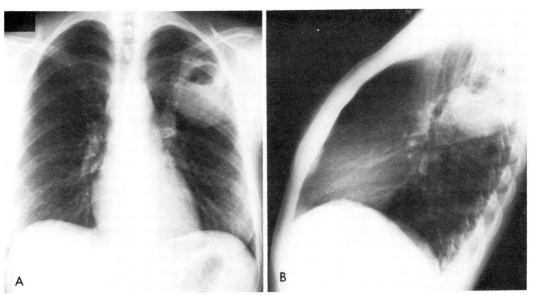

A

B

Figure 5–4. Abscess, left upper lobe, with cavitation. This large pyogenic abscess with cavitation is more likely benign or inflammatory than malignant, because the inner wall of the cavity is smooth and the upper margin is thin (see Chapter 7). Note also that the mass, on the lateral view (B), bulges the major fissure inferiorly.

CHAPTER 6

HYPERLUCENCY AND CHRONIC OBSTRUCTIVE PULMONARY DISEASE

Increased lucency in one or both lungs or in parts of one or both lungs is a common radiographic finding. Its causes include the following:

1. Technical factors. The position of the x-ray tube in relation to a grid or the position of the patient in relation to the film cassette can cause a nonuniform radiation distribution. This can result in unilateral lucency or density of a lung.
2. Abnormalities of the chest wall. Soft tissue asymmetry is another frequent cause of relative hyperlucency. Most often this is seen after surgery, especially a mastectomy (Fig. 1–12).
3. Air trapping
   a. Due to a ball valve mechanism in a major bronchus (Fig. 6–1). This can be caused by an intrinsic or extrinsic neoplasm, enlarged lymph nodes, a foreign body, a broncholith or mucosal thickening by granulomatous disease or amyloid.
   b. Asthma, bronchitis and cystic fibrosis can cause local or diffuse air trapping (Fig. 6–2).
   c. Inflammatory disease of the small airways, as seen in bronchiolitis obliterans. This may be local or diffuse.
   d. Patchy or diffuse destruction of the pulmonary parenchyma due to emphysema (Fig. 6–3).
4. Decreased vascularity
   a. Secondary to parenchymal or airway disease (Fig. 6–4).
   b. Pulmonary embolism.
   c. Pulmonary arterial hypertension (central vessels large, peripheral vessels small or inapparent).
   d. Primary or secondary neoplasm involving the pulmonary arteries.
   e. Congenital cardiovascular or bronchial anomalies.
5. Bullae, blebs and pneumatoceles (Fig. 6–5)
6. Pneumothorax
7. Regions of compensatory emphysema due to volume loss in an adjacent lobe(s)

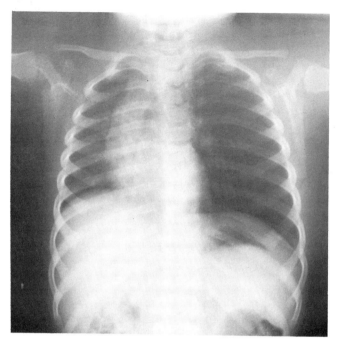

Figure 6–1. Obstructive emphysema because of foreign body in left mainstem bronchus. This child aspirated a peanut. Because the peanut is obstructing outflow of air more than it is obstructing inflow ("ball valve mechanism"), air trapping has resulted. The left lung is overdistended, the left hemidiaphragm is depressed and the mediastinum is shifted toward the right.

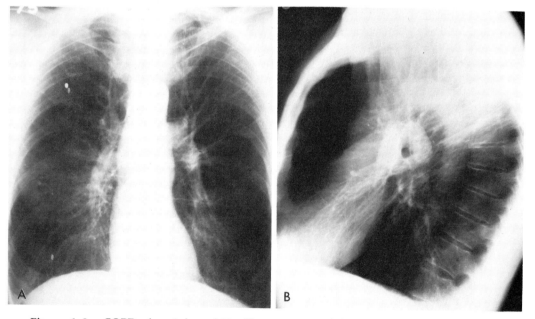

Figure 6–2. COPD, chronic bronchitis. Hyperaeration of the lungs is obvious on both frontal (A) and lateral (B) films. The most distinctive finding, flattening of the hemidiaphragms, is especially obvious on the lateral view. There is no evidence for significant decreased vascularity in the lung fields.

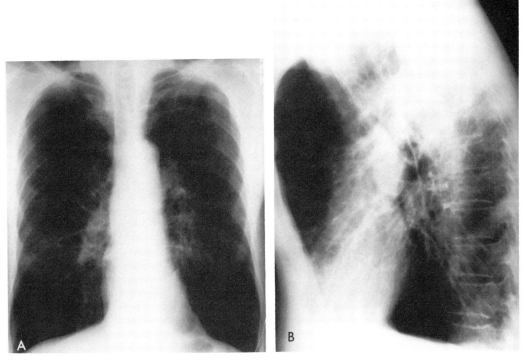

Figure 6–3. COPD, emphysema. As in Figure 6–2, hyperexpansion is evident on both frontal (*A*) and lateral (*B*) films. Flattened hemidiaphragms are again obvious. In contrast to chronic bronchitis, however, pulmonary vascularity is diminished bilaterally, especially at the periphery of the lung fields. This finding correlates only moderately well with pulmonary-function-test evidence of emphysema.

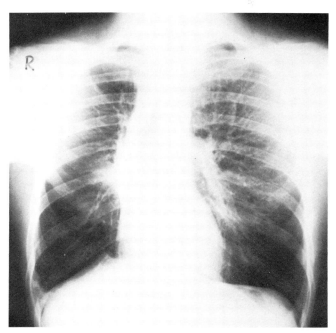

Figure 6–4. Swyer-James-McCloud syndrome. Air trapping is present in both lower lobes, and blood flow is diminished to both lower lobes and the right upper lobe. The left upper lobe is the only normal lobe in this case and is the only well-vascularized region. In this syndrome, an early childhood infection causes bronchiolitis obliterans and poor pulmonary arterial development in one or more lobes of lung. The affected lobes show diminished vascularity but may be normal or underventilated or show air trapping.

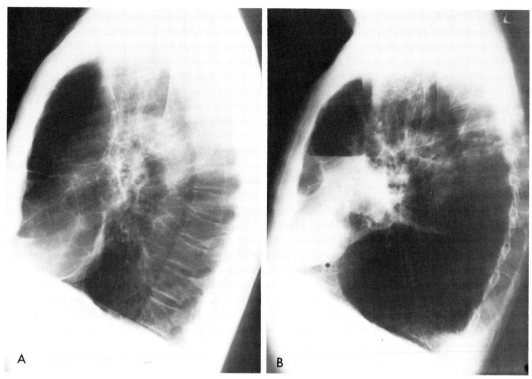

Figure 6–5. Bullous emphysema, lateral views. Large bullae are evident, especially in the anterior lung field on a routine lateral film (*A*). Pulmonary infection later developed in this patient, causing exudate within the bullae as well as free pleural effusion (*B*).

The radiographic diagnosis of chronic obstructive lung disease (chronic bronchitis, emphysema, asthma) is possible in approximately half the people who have significant disease (Figs. 6–2 and 6–3). Most commonly this is manifest radiographically as diffuse air trapping. Increase in the total volume of the lungs may be judged by the low, flat configuration of the diaphragm, increased AP diameter and increased retrosternal lucency. Such patients may also have areas of decreased vascularity and bullae, which are reliable signs of severe parenchymal destruction due to COPD. Bullae and blebs (Fig. 6–5) may be seen in patients who do not have generalized obstructive lung disease, but multiple bullae usually are associated with severe emphysema. When emphysematous changes are predominantly in the lower lung fields, especially in a young person, alpha I antitrypsin deficiency disease should always be considered as a possible cause.

CHAPTER 7

HOLES IN THE LUNG

THIN-WALLED HOLES

Bullae, blebs and cysts are difficult to distinguish from one another and often are not clinically important unless they are due to cystic bronchiectasis or become secondarily infected. If infected, the wall of the "hole" usually becomes thicker and a fluid level may be seen (Fig. 6–5). Thin-walled lesions may be due to congenital conditions, emphysema, previous infection, trauma or dilated destroyed airways (cystic bronchiectasis) (Figs. 7–1 and 7–2).

CAVITIES

The term "cavity" implies destruction of the pulmonary parenchyma, with necrosis and discharge of material into bronchi. Typically the underlying disease process is of grave clinical concern. Common causes include the following:

1. Infection: bacterial pneumonia, aspiration lung abscess, septic emboli (Fig. 7–3), tuberculosis and other granulomatous infections (Fig. 7–4), various parasitic diseases (especially amebiasis, hydatid disease, paragonimiasis).
2. Neoplasm: primary or metastatic disease, particularly of an epidermoid cell type (Fig. 7–5); Hodgkin's disease.
3. Vasculitis and/or collagen disease: Wegener's granulomatosis, lymphomatoid granulomatosis and rheumatoid lung.

The character of the wall of a cavitary lesion is helpful in the differential diagnosis of these lesions. Cavities caused by malignant disease tend to have nodular and irregular inner walls, although the outer walls may be sharply or poorly defined (Fig. 7–5). Benign and inflammatory cavities usually have smooth inner walls (Figs. 7–3 and 7–4). In addition, the thicker the wall of a cavity, the more likely malignancy becomes, except in the case of cavities that have arisen very rapidly (over a few days), in which case the cavity is usually traumatic or infectious in origin.

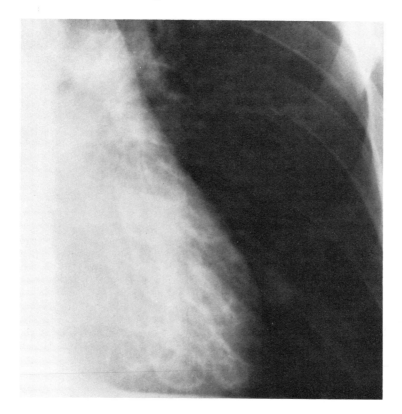

Figure 7–1. Cystic bronchiectasis, left lower lobe. Multiple thin-walled cysts here represent dilated small bronchi that have become markedly distended by chronic inflammation. The location of these lesions along the bronchial pathways is often difficult to differentiate from randomly located cavities.

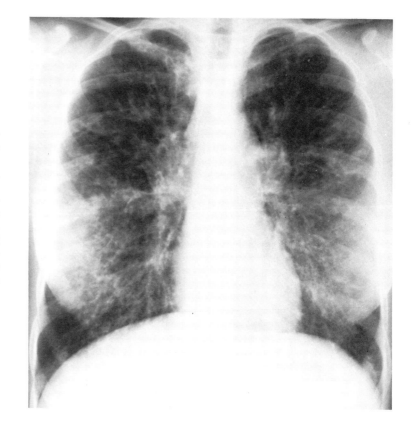

Figure 7–2. Severe cystic bronchiectasis in cystic fibrosis. An interstitial pattern, caused by scarring from many previous pneumonias, is mixed with cystic bronchiectasis, as previously defined in Figure 7–1. Typically, the bronchiectasis of cystic fibrosis is most prominent in the upper lung fields (in this case especially the right upper lung field).

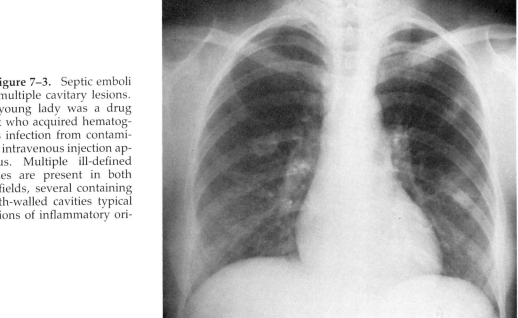

Figure 7–3. Septic emboli with multiple cavitary lesions. This young lady was a drug addict who acquired hematogenous infection from contaminated intravenous injection apparatus. Multiple ill-defined nodules are present in both lung fields, several containing smooth-walled cavities typical of lesions of inflammatory origin.

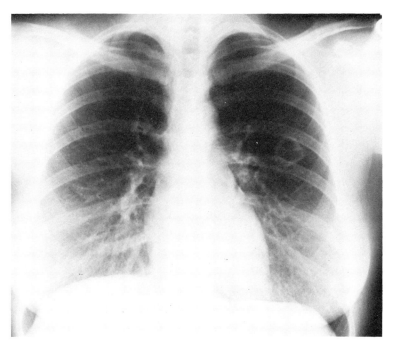

Figure 7–4. Coccidioidomycosis with cavitary mass. This fungal disease, common in the southwestern region of the United States, is characteristically manifest as smooth, thin-walled cavities. The smooth inner wall is most distinctive for the nonmalignant origin of such a cavity.

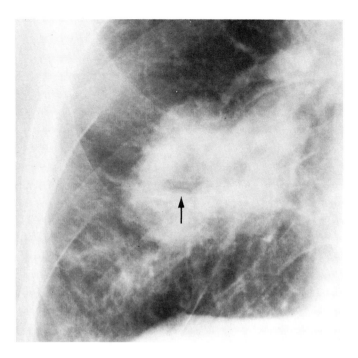

Figure 7–5. Malignant cavitary mass of squamous bronchogenic carcinoma. This closeup view of the right lower lobe shows a mass with an indistinct central cavity and an air fluid level (arrow). The nodular character of the inner wall and the overall wall thickness strongly suggest the malignant nature of this necrotic lesion.

CHAPTER 8

PERIPHERAL PULMONARY LESIONS

Pulmonary infiltrates may be diffuse, involving all of both lung fields, or localized. Localized lesions can be segmental if they involve specific bronchopulmonary segments or lobes. Those localized lesions that are nonsegmental include the perihilar distribution of pulmonary edema, the lower lung field distribution of most collagen diseases and asbestosis, and the upper lung field distribution of most granulomatous diseases, such as tuberculosis.

Peripheral distribution of nonsegmental localized disease is relatively unusual and thus suggests certain specific diagnoses, depending upon the specific portion of the periphery that is primarily involved.

APICAL ABNORMALITIES

1. Capping. One, or more commonly both, of the lung apices may have a thin, regular rim of increased density. This is usually termed "apical capping." Pathologically, fibrotic lung and perhaps slightly thickened pleura are found. There are no clinical consequences of this situation, and its cause is uncertain. A large percentage of chest radiographs, particularly in older individuals, show this finding.

2. Scars. Irregular densities due to scarring are common in the lung apices (Fig. 8–1). Often these can be traced to previous granulomatous infection.

3. Granulomatous Infection. The reactivation or chronic form of granulomatous infection typically involves the apices. Nodularity, irregular scarring, poorly defined consolidation, volume loss, irregular cyst formation and calcification are all common (Fig. 8–2).

4. Cancer. Carcinoma of the lung often arises in the apex. If it invades the pleura and chest wall, it is called a Pancoast or superior sulcus tumor (Fig. 8–3). Clinically these patients have local and/or referred pain and perhaps a Horner's syndrome. Many show radiographic evidence of local bone destruction in addition to an apical mass.

5. Blebs. Blebs or bullae are common in the apices, and careful inspection will often reveal part of their margins (Fig. 8–1). These are often not associated with diffuse pulmonary emphysema. They may cause spontaneous pneumothorax.

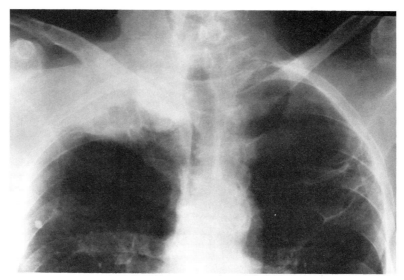

Figure 8–1. Right apical scarring of old granulomatous disease. The irregularity of the right apical density and the presence of irregular cystic spaces and linear densities distinguish this abnormality from "apical capping." A calcified granuloma is noted lower in the periphery of the right lung field and several linear scars are also noted in the left upper lung field. The left apex contains a large emphysematous bleb that is somewhat expansile.

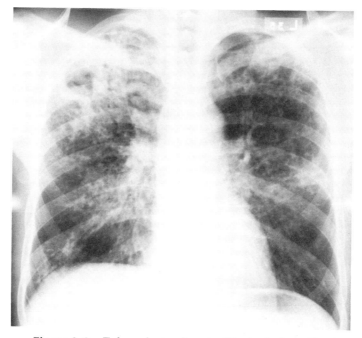

Figure 8–2. Tuberculosis, chronic. The typical predilection of tuberculosis for the upper lung field is manifest by irregular densities, masses and a large cavity in the right upper lung field. The hazy quality of the infiltration suggests activity of the granulomatous disease.

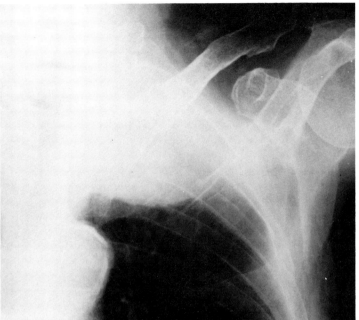

Figure 8–3. Bronchogenic carcinoma, Pancoast type, left apex. This homogeneous density in the left apex was found to invade the chest wall and, although not seen clearly here, there was erosion of the third left posterior rib. Distinct differences between such a tumor and inflammatory or fibrotic disease are often not evident.

6. **Radiation Fibrosis.** Radiation often produces a characteristic band of increased density in the apex several months after administration using a supraclavicular port. Similar findings may be seen along the mediastinum and along the lateral lung margins after appropriate radiation ports such as a "mantle" configuration (Fig. 8–4). Unlike acute radiation pneumonia, which usually causes cough, fever and even cyanosis, these patients are typically asymptomatic unless a large volume of lung is involved. A pulmonary infiltrate with a sharp border that is not a recognizable fissure should always suggest radiation pneumonia or fibrosis as a possible cause.

7. **Artifacts.** Artifacts often overlie the lung apices. Commonly this is jewelry, an article of clothing or hair.

LATERAL LUNG FIELDS

Occasionally, infectious pneumonia (often pneumococcal) or aspiration pneumonia is localized to the periphery of a lateral lung field. Such consolidation often has an axillary distribution involving either a separate segment of the upper lobe or parts of the anterior and posterior segments (Fig. 8–5). Presumably, secretions are aspirated and pooled in these areas with the patient lying on his side. A very similar appearance also occurs in pulmonary embolism and infarction. Wedge-shaped peripheral regions of consolidation represent hemorrhage and edema in an area deprived of pulmonary arterial flow. Peripheral interstitial infiltration may suggest allergic disease origin but is usually a nonspecific finding (Fig. 8–6).

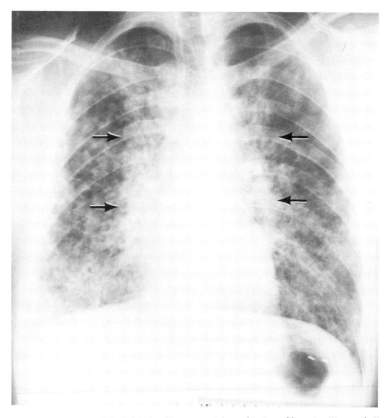

Figure 8–4. Hodgkin's disease with radiation fibrosis ("mantle" pattern) and superimposed viral pneumonia. The nodular pattern in this patient's lung fields was found on autopsy to be secondary to both metastatic Hodgkin's disease and viral pneumonia with hemorrhage. The consolidated areas on either side of the mediastinum are demarcated from the surrounding lung by a sharp border (arrows), which was the radiation port. Radiation fibrosis was pathologically demonstrated in this region (AFIP negative #75–11384).

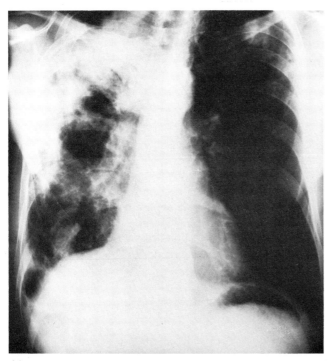

Figure 8–5. Pneumonia, necrotizing, right upper lobe. Irregular consolidation here involves the periphery of the right upper lung field, including the pleura. There is also right volume loss with an elevated hemidiaphragm. Aspiration was probably responsible for this distribution in this patient.

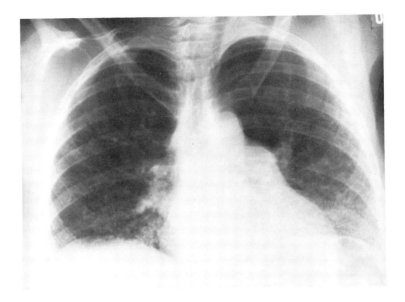

Figure 8–6. Bibasilar and peripheral interstitial infiltration, cause unknown. Marked volume loss is present, in addition to a mild interstitial infiltrate. Diffuse interstitial pneumonitis (usual interstitial pneumonitis) was found at autopsy with no evident cause. Such nonspecific cases with predominantly peripheral distribution sometimes suggest allergic etiologies.

BASAL ABNORMALITIES

Acute basal consolidation is usually due to pneumonia or aspiration. Chronic basilar interstitial infiltration should suggest several possibilities, especially chronic aspiration, lymphangitic metastatic disease, asbestosis, idiopathic fibrosis or fibrosis associated with collagen disease (particularly scleroderma, rheumatoid disease, or a mixed connective tissue disorder) (Figs. 8–6 and 8–7). Bronchiectasis, while not a cause of a true interstitial infiltrate, may have an appearance resembling bibasilar interstitial infiltration.

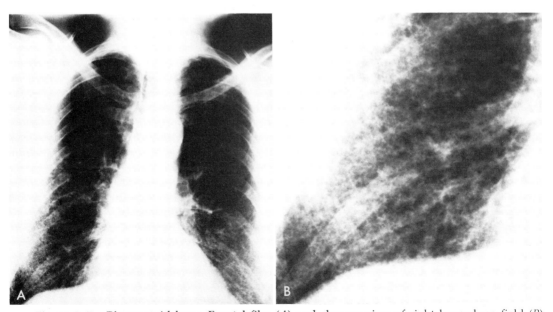

Figure 8–7. Rheumatoid lung. Frontal film (*A*) and closeup view of right lower lung field (*B*) show an interstitial pattern most prevalent at the base of the periphery of the lung fields. This appearance is nonspecific, but its causes are so varied that the clinical history is usually extremely helpful in differential diagnosis.

CHAPTER 9

HILAR ENLARGEMENT

The hila are the roots of the lungs where the pulmonary arteries and bronchi emerge. In the normal person most of the radiographic density is due to the central pulmonary arteries. Air outlines the major bronchi. The many lymph nodes in the hila are not detected unless they are enlarged.

Understanding the hilar shadows is greatly simplified by recalling a few important anatomic facts. The pulmonary arteries and bronchi lie superior and slightly anterior to the confluence of the pulmonary veins on each side. On the left side, the pulmonary artery crosses over the left upper lobe bronchus and descends posterior to the bronchi in the left lower lobe. The right pulmonary artery descends anterior to the bronchus intermedius and is thus lower and more anterior than the left pulmonary artery. This relationship is easily seen on the lateral view, on which the two pulmonary arteries and the two upper lobe bronchi (seen on end as round lucencies) are often identifiable (Fig. 9–1).

BILATERAL HILAR ENLARGEMENT

Bilateral hilar enlargement is typically due to either enlargement of the central pulmonary arteries or lymphadenopathy.

VASCULAR DILATATION

There is considerable normal variation in the size of the main pulmonary arteries. Prominence of the hila is typically noted in cases of pregnancy and obesity and on hypoventilatory films.

Significant enlargement of the major pulmonary arteries is almost invariably due to pulmonary arterial hypertension (Fig. 9–2). Clues to the vascular nature of the enlarged hila are the contour (typically it is round and/or tubular) and the frequent presence of coexistent abnormalities of medium-sized and peripheral pulmonary arteries.

Common causes of pulmonary hypertension with enlarged hila are congestive heart failure, mitral valve disease (particularly stenosis), left to right shunts, diffuse pulmonary parenchymal disease (emphysema, sarcoidosis, pulmonary fibrosis and many others less common), primary small vessel disease, idiopathic and pulmonary embolism (massive or recurrent).

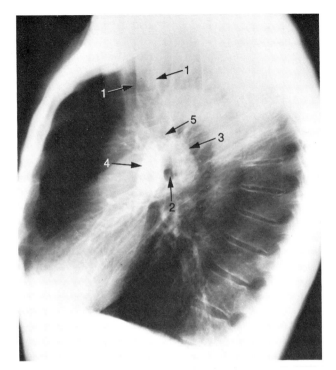

Figure 9–1. Lateral chest film demonstrating hilar anatomy. The pulmonary arteries are slightly enlarged in this patient with COPD. For orientation, the uppermost arrows denote the trachea. This lucency can be followed inferiorly to the left upper lobe bronchus seen on end (arrow 2). The left pulmonary artery (arrow 3) is above and posterior to this bronchus. The right pulmonary artery (arrow 4) is anterior. The right upper lobe bronchus (arrow 5) is not clearly seen because of the slight enlargement of the pulmonary arteries in this case.

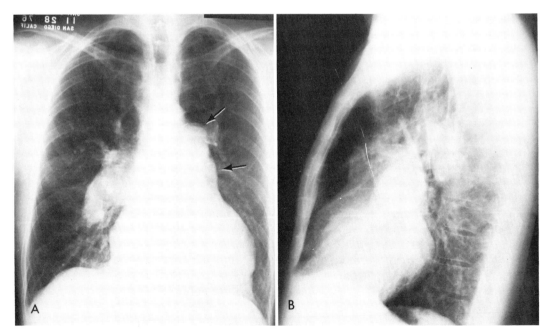

Figure 9–2. Pulmonary arterial hypertension, chronic. Marked enlargement of the pulmonary arteries with calcification of their walls is seen on both frontal (A) and lateral (B) views. On the frontal view (A) the left pulmonary artery (upper arrow) nearly obscures the aortic arch. The main pulmonary artery (lower arrow) is also markedly enlarged. The rounded, bulbous shape of the pulmonary arteries on the left view (B) should be compared to the normal shape seen in Figure 9–1.

NODAL

Clues to lymphadenopathy include a lobulated contour of the enlarged hilum (Fig. 9–3) and evidence of mediastinal lymphadenopathy, particularly in the right paratracheal and aorto-pulmonary window region.

Common causes include sarcoidosis, infectious granulomatous disease, neoplasm (especially lymphoma), and metastatic carcinoma (often from lung, breast, testes, kidney). Diffuse or patchy calcification in hilar lymph nodes is a reliable indication that the etiology is previous granulomatous disease (infectious or noninfectious such as silicosis), and usually no further evaluation is necessary. Symmetric hilar (often accompanied by paratracheal) lymphadenopathy in an asymptomatic young adult is almost always due to sarcoidosis.

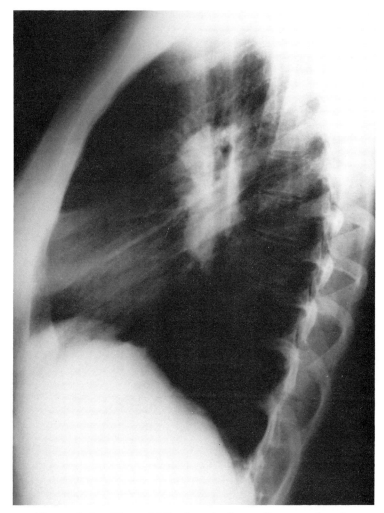

Figure 9–3. Bilateral hilar lymphadenopathy secondary to sarcoidosis. Nodular enlargement of the hilum with normal pulmonary vascularity is evident on this lateral film. The normal contours of the pulmonary arteries are obscured by the enlarged lymph nodes surrounding them.

UNILATERAL HILAR ENLARGEMENT

1. Vascular: idiopathic, pulmonary embolism, pulmonic stenosis (left side only), aneurysm.
2. Neoplasm: usually a primary bronchogenic carcinoma.
3. Lymphadenopathy: same differential diagnosis as with bilateral lymphadenopathy except that sarcoidosis is rarely unilateral.

CHAPTER **10**

MEDIASTINAL DISEASE

The various structures of the mediastinum are principally of soft tissue density and, therefore, are difficult to separate from one another. Distinguishing normal mediastinal width from pathological enlargement can be difficult. Poor inspiration or rotation of the patient's film will cause diffuse widening of the mediastinal shadow. Mediastinal masses are only visualized if they displace or obscure the pleural interface between mediastinum and air-containing lung. The apparent lateral boundaries of the mediastinum on the frontal view represent only the most lateral portions of the pleura reflecting over the mediastinal structures. Detection of subtle mediastinal abnormalities requires thorough knowledge of the location and appearance of the pleural interface as it courses over the structures of the mediastinum.

PNEUMOMEDIASTINUM

Linear lucencies due to air collections are found with pneumomediastinum (Fig. 10–1). Pneumomediastinum can be due to surgery, a penetrating wound, leakage from the esophagus or major airways, or hyperbaric damage to the pulmonary parenchyma, with air traveling along the bronchovascular bundles back into the mediastinum. This latter condition is seen in acute asthma, after severe coughing episodes and in patients on respirators (especially if PEEP is used).

DIFFUSE WIDENING

CHRONIC OR SLOWLY CHANGING

Most often chronic mediastinal widening is of no clinical concern and is due to tortuous atherosclerotic great vessels (Fig. 10–2). Occasionally vascular anomalies also cause diffuse widening.

Mediastinal fat in abnormally large quantity can be seen in obesity, steroid therapy or Cushing's syndrome. Other common causes of gradual widening are indistinguishable and include neoplasm, aneurysm, esophageal dilatation (most marked and common with achalasia), chronic granulomatous infection (most typically seen in histoplasmosis, where there can be associated calcification, or the syndrome of fibrosing mediastinitis) and surgery (particularly esophageal bypass and coronary artery bypass) (Fig. 10–3).

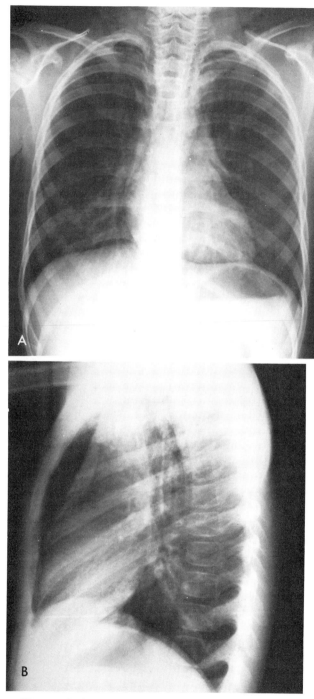

Figure 10–1. Pneumomediastinum and subcutaneous emphysema secondary to asthma. Vertical linear lucencies are seen on both frontal (A) and lateral (B) films separating and surrounding the normal structures of the mediastinum. The lucencies extend superiorly into the neck.

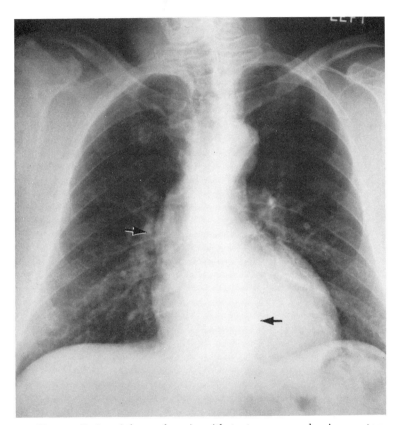

Figure 10–2. Atherosclerosis with tortuous vessels. A very tortuous, atherosclerotic thoracic aorta bulges to the right (arrow) in its ascending portion and again on the left (lower arrow) behind the heart in its descending portion. A bulging, tortuous brachiocephalic artery is also noted just behind the medial portion of the right clavicle.

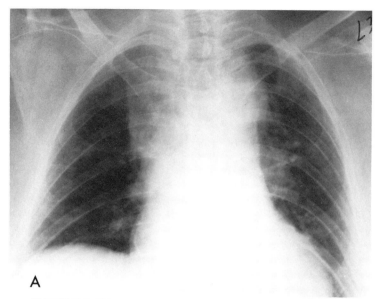

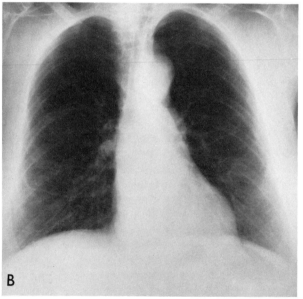

Figure 10–3. Postsurgical mediastinal widening secondary to fibrosing hemorrhage. Marked diffuse widening of the mediastinum is obvious on the postoperative view (*A*). A preoperative film (*B*) shows the normal contour of the mediastinum, save for a tortuous, atherosclerotic aorta.

ACUTE

Any fluid material can acutely widen the mediastinum. The resulting appearance is identical to that of gradual widening (Fig. 10–3). Clear fluid is usually from an iatrogenic source, particularly a malpositioned CVP line. Mediastinal edema is rare. Bleeding into the mediastinum is usually due to trauma or surgery. Patients who are on anticoagulants or who have a bleeding diathesis, a leaking aneurysm or a neoplasm may hemorrhage into the mediastinum spontaneously.

Dissecting aneurysm of the aorta causes acute widening without extravascular accumulation of blood in some patients.

Pus may accumulate after a penetrating injury or surgery, dissect down from a neck abscess, or collect after perforation of the esophagus or trachea. Chyle leaks from the thoracic duct into the mediastinum and/or pleural space from congenital anomalies of the lymphatic system. Neoplasm or trauma can also disrupt the thoracic duct.

LOCAL ABNORMALITIES

Local mediastinal abnormalities are commonly seen with lymphadenopathy, neoplasm, aneurysm, vascular anomaly (e.g., coarctation of the aorta), hiatus hernia and esophageal disease, including diverticulum and neoplasm.

Lymphadenopathy frequently has a characteristic lobulated contour. Involvement of the paratracheal area and/or hila is also common (Fig. 10–4).

Aneurysms and vascular anomalies have characteristic locations in continuity with other vascular structures (Fig. 10–5). A calcific rim may be a clue to vascular origin but may also occur in cysts and even malignant cystic masses.

Hiatus hernia and esophageal diverticulum often contain air with or without a fluid level (Fig. 10–6). Small amounts of air are often seen in a normal esophagus, but a large amount suggests esophageal obstruction.

The mediastinum can be divided into compartments in many different ways. The most useful subdivisions for radiologists are anterior, middle and posterior, with the upper portion of each subdivision (above the top of the aortic arch) often referred to as the "superior" mediastinum. The anterior and middle mediastinum are divided by a line drawn through the anterior wall of the trachea and the posterior border of the heart; this allows all masses of the heart and pericardium to be included as anterior mediastinal masses. The middle mediastinum extends from this line to the front of the vertebral bodies as seen on the lateral view. Masses centered behind the front of the vertebral bodies are considered posterior. It is best to consider the superior mediastinum as a superior continuation of each of the other three compartments.

Location of a mediastinal mass is often a clue to etiology. A large mass extending from the neck into the mediastinum, deviating the trachea to either side and causing a soft tissue density behind the trachea on the lateral film, is almost always an enlarged thyroid, often a goiter (Fig. 10–7). Anterior mediastinal masses are most commonly thymoma (or thymus) (Fig. 10–8), teratoma or lymphoma. A low anterior mass is often a pericardial cyst (Fig. 10–9). Middle mediastinal masses often are due to nodes or benign cysts. Neoplasms (usually benign) of neural origin are the dominant cause of purely posterior mediastinal masses (Fig. 10–10).

Lymphadenopathy and malignancy may be seen anywhere in the mediastinum. Occasionally adjacent bony destruction is the clue to a malignant process. Less frequently benign disease, such as aortic aneurysm or benign neural tumors, causes adjacent bony destruction by pressure erosion. In these cases, the margin of bone destruction is usually well defined or sclerotic, indicating the indolent nature of the disease process.

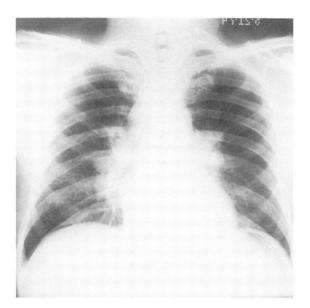

Figure 10–4. Mediastinal and hilar lymphadenopathy secondary to sarcoidosis. In addition to diffuse, nodular widening of the mediastinum, there is marked bilateral hilar lymphadenopathy, which is typical of sarcoidosis.

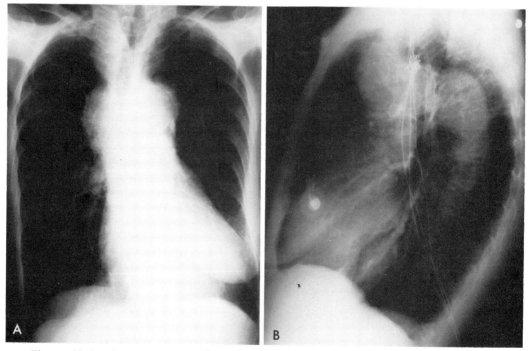

Figure 10–5. Aneurysm, ascending aorta. On the frontal film (A) the bulge of the right mediastinum opposite the aortic knob is a localized aneurysm of unknown origin. A tortuous brachiocephalic artery and calcification of the aortic knob are also evident on the frontal film. The lateral film (B) shows the anterior location of the aneurysm, with minimal posterior displacement of the trachea. This patient also has cardiomegaly and a right mastectomy.

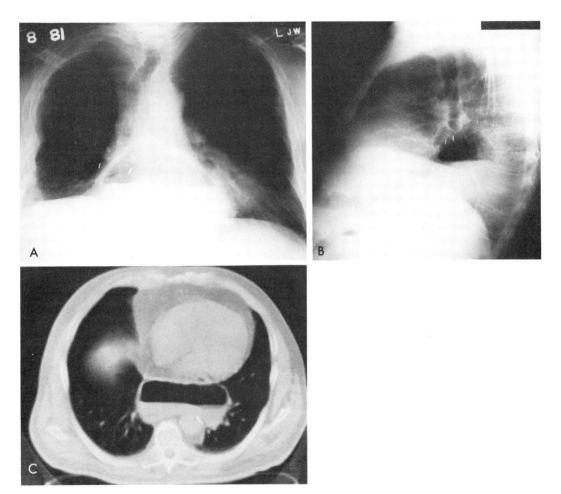

Figure 10–6. Hiatal hernia. A large air-containing mass with an air fluid level is seen on the frontal view (*A*) and in the middle mediastinum on the lateral view (*B*). A CT cross section (*C*) also shows the air fluid level behind the heart and anterior to the aorta with the patient lying supine. The hazy density in the right lung field is the uppermost portion of the right hemidiaphragm.

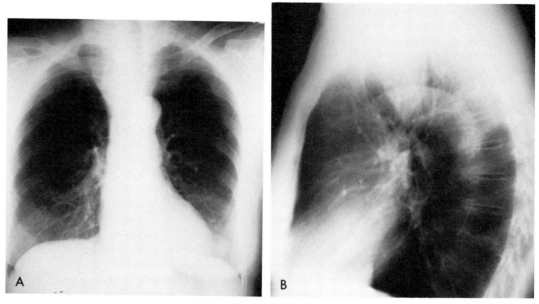

Figure 10–7. Diffuse thyroid enlargement, goiter. A mass in the superior mediastinum, widening the mediastinum above the aorta on the frontal view (A) and deviating the trachea anteriorly on the lateral view (B), is evident. On the frontal view (A) the trachea is also deviated slightly to the left.

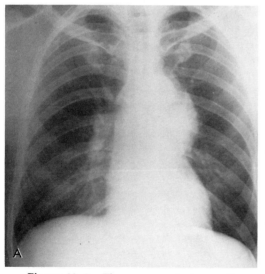

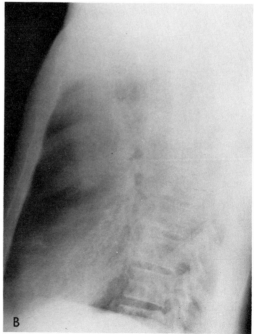

Figure 10–8. Thymoma, anterior mediastinum. On the frontal view (A) a large mass above the left heart border is seen. The anterior location is evident on the lateral view (B), nearly filling the clear space superior to the heart.

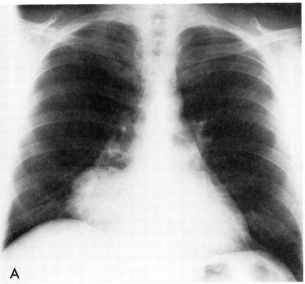

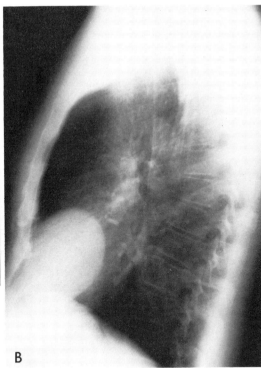

Figure 10–9. Pericardial cyst, anterior mediastinum. Frontal (*A*) and lateral (*B*) views show a very sharply bordered mass far anterior in the right cardiophrenic angle. This is the most common location and appearance for a pericardial cyst.

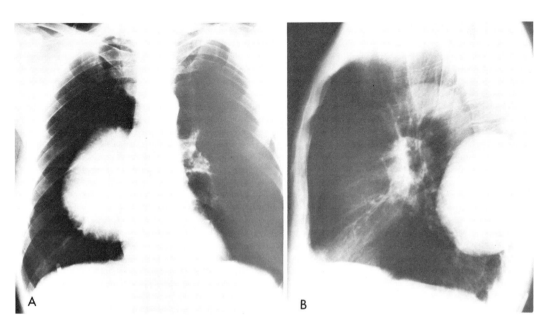

Figure 10–10. Neurilemoma (schwannoma), posterior mediastinum. This unusually large neural tumor is evident on frontal (*A*) and lateral (*B*) views. The sharp borders are typical, but the large size is unusual for this diagnosis.

CHAPTER 11

THE DIAPHRAGM

Slight to moderate elevation and/or irrregularity of the diaphragm is usually a normal variant. A good practical principle is to ignore such a finding unless there is definite interval change on the radiographs or corresponding symptoms are present.

ELEVATION

Elevation of the hemidiaphragm is most often due to a normal variant or eventration.

Eventration of the diaphragm is thinning and weakness of the normal muscle. Common sites are the following:

1. Anteromedially on the right.
2. Posterolaterally on either side. This may be a small or incomplete Bochdalek hernia (Fig. 11–1).

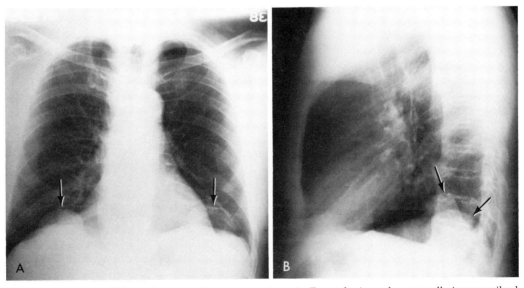

Figure 11–1. Bilateral eventrations, posterior. *A,* Frontal view shows well-circumscribed eventrations of both hemidiaphragms, with the normal crest of each diaphragm seen through the shadow of the eventration. *B,* The lateral view shows posterior location, with the eventration of the left hemidiaphragm (upper arrow) projecting slightly higher than the larger eventration of the right hemidiaphragm (lower arrow). The fact that the right hemidiaphragm projects more posteriorly than the left hemidiaphragm is clearly seen by comparing the size of the ribs where they turn; the more posterior ribs are more magnified because they are farther from the film on this left lateral projection.

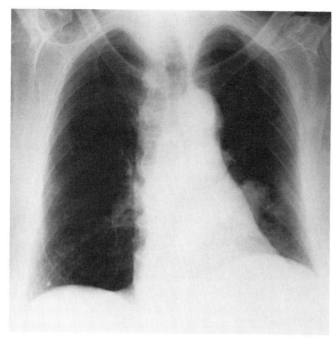

Figure 11–2. Paralysis, left hemidiaphragm, secondary to bronchogenic carcinoma. In this case, a bronchogenic carcinoma, seen just behind the mid left heart border, has invaded the mediastinum adjacent to the heart and disrupted phrenic nerve function. The resulting paralysis of the left hemidiaphragm is identical to eventration of the entire left hemidiaphragm on the inspiratory frontal view.

3. The entire left hemidiaphragm. This is difficult to distinguish from paralysis (Fig. 11–2). Frequently in this form of eventration the posterior muscle fibers are intact, so that fluoroscopy reveals paradoxical movement or no movement of the large anterior portion of the left hemidiaphragm but normal movement of the most posterior portion.

Other common causes of diaphragmatic elevation include paralysis (Fig. 11–3), splinting due to a nearby fracture or other cause of local pain, subdiaphragmatic disease (especially an abscess) (Figs. 11–4 and 11–5), pneumonia, pulmonary embolism, subjacent abdominal organomegaly (Fig. 11–6). Subpulmonic pleural effusion (Chapter 12) is the most common cause of apparent (but not real) diaphragmatic elevation.

HERNIAS

Herniation through the esophageal hiatus usually involves part of the stomach (Fig. 10–6). Occasionally the entire stomach, omentum or even other abdominal viscera may herniate through this hiatus. Plain radiographs of the chest frequently show a retrocardiac density, which may have a fluid level.

Two forms of congenital herniation are common. Anteromedially (usually on the right) omentum or bowel can herniate through the foramen of Morgagni. These hernias are usually asymptomatic. Bochdalek hernias occur posterolaterally on either side (remember: *B* for back!). Occasionally massive herniation of abdominal contents into the chest occurs through such a hernia (Fig. 11–7). This can be fatal in an infant.

Post-traumatic hernias can be due to blunt or penetrating trauma. They are also occasionally seen after surgery that violates the diaphragm. These hernias usually occur on the left, since the liver protects the right hemidiaphragm and blocks small organs from herniating upward.

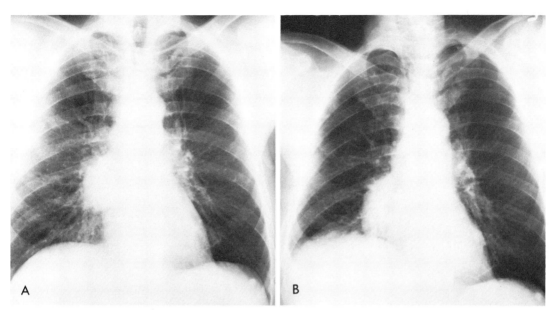

Figure 11–3. Paralysis, right hemidiaphragm, secondary to bronchogenic carcinoma. Upon initial presentation with a squamous bronchogenic carcinoma of the right hilum, diaphragmatic position and appearance were normal (*A*). As the mass enlarged, it disrupted function of the right phrenic nerve, resulting in elevation of the right hemidiaphragm (*B*) with marked volume loss in the right lower lung field. The lower lobe volume loss is responsible for the haziness of the diaphragm on the later film (*B*).

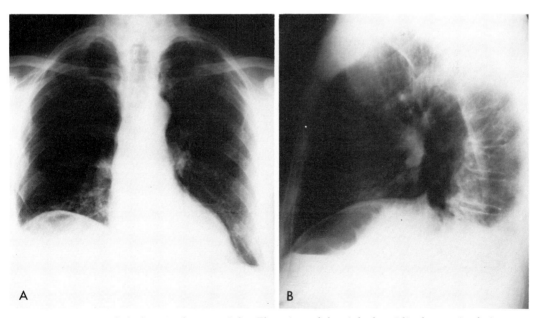

Figure 11–4. Subphrenic abscess, right. Elevation of the right hemidiaphragm is obvious on both frontal (*A*) and lateral (*B*) views. A large air lucency is noted beneath the hemidiaphragm on both views and shows an air fluid level on the lateral view (*B*). A right pleural effusion is also evident. With the exception of the effusion, the appearance here is not definitely abnormal, as the hepatic flexure of colon may be interposed between liver and diaphragm in normal individuals, mimicking the appearance of an air-containing subphrenic abscess.

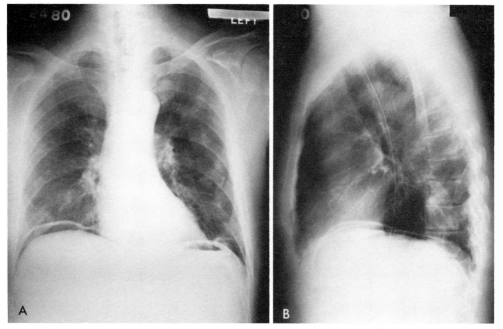

Figure 11–5. Pneumoperitoneum. Air is interposed between liver and lower diaphrag-matic surface on both frontal (*A*) and lateral (*B*) views. The air lucency beneath the left hemidiaphragm is the normal stomach bubble. Useful signs in excluding interposition of colon (see Fig. 11–4) include the smooth upper border of the liver, the lack of haustral markings within the lucency of air, and the length of the lucency on both frontal and lateral views.

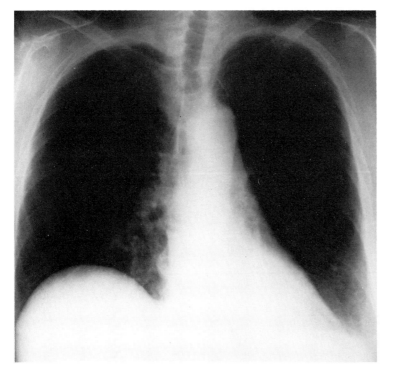

Figure 11–6. Elevation, right hemidiaphragm, secondary to liver enlargement. There are no roentgenographic hints by which this elevated right hemidiaphragm could be distinguished from a large eventration or from a subpulmonic right effusion. Fluoroscopy, CT or a liver radiopharmaceutical scan could be used for differential diagnosis.

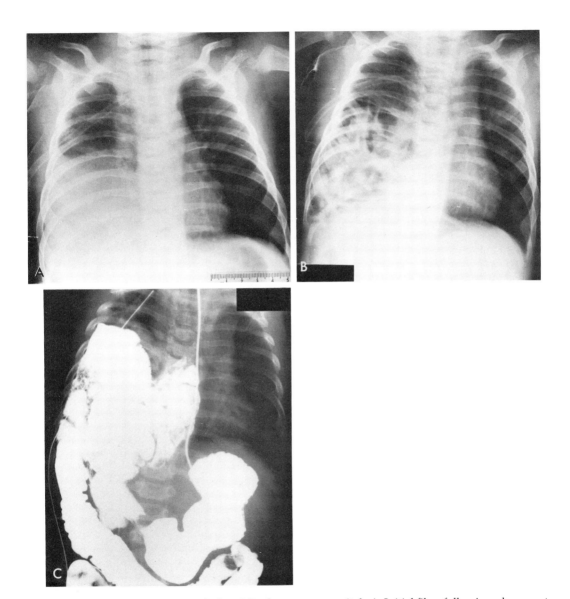

Figure 11–7. Herniation, right hemidiaphragm, congenital. *A,* Initial film, following placement of right chest tube for presumed right pleural effusion, shows increased density in right lower lung field and no apparent diaphragmatic surface. *B,* A subsequent film shows irregular air lucencies, which could represent cystic lung lesions but in fact represent bowel air. Note the suggestion of haustral markings in the uppermost lucencies. *C,* Barium swallow shows marked herniation of bowel loops, now filled with barium, into the right hemithorax (AFIP negative #76–4678).

CHAPTER 12

PLEURAL DISEASE

Pleural abnormalities are recognizable because of their typical location and configuration. Peripheral location or continuity with a fissure aids in recognition of an extraparenchymal process. Pleural or extrapleural lesions characteristically have an elliptical or some other noncircular shape because their expansion is not equal in all directions and the pressure of the lung flattens the lesion toward the periphery (Fig. 12–1).

THICKENING

Pleural thickening and adhesions (tenting) are usually chronic and due to scarring from some previous insult such as infection, trauma or asbestos exposure. They can be local or diffuse. An acute inflammatory process can cause localized pleural thickening. Asbestos exposure is an important cause of pleural plaques that are usually bilateral and may be calcified (Fig. 12–2). Calcification of the diaphragm can also occur with asbestos exposure and is virtually always caused by asbestos (occasionally talc). The identification of previous asbestos exposure is important because of the carcinogenicity associated with such exposure.

Extrapleural fat mimics pleural thickening. Its typically smooth, symmetric contour and apical or axillary distribution in a patient who is obese or on steroids or who has Cushing's disease usually allows recognition.

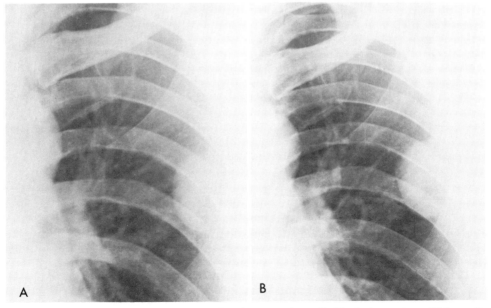

Figure 12–1. Pleural lipoma. *A,* Inspiratory view. *B,* Expiratory view. This well-circumscribed elliptical mass indents the lateral portion of the lung from its origin on the pleural surface. The change in shape during respiration is distinct for soft pleural masses, especially lipomas. Note that the greater aeration of lung in the inspiratory view (*A*) flattens the lesions toward the chest wall in comparison to the expiratory view (*B*) (AFIP negative #55–4271).

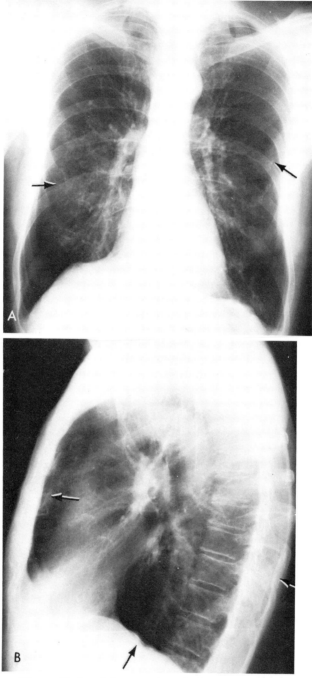

Figure 12–2. Asbestos pleural plaques and calcification. *A,* Frontal view of this construction worker with a long history of asbestos exposure shows extremely minimal changes other than the hyperexpansion of emphysema; hazy densities (arrows) are actually pleural calcifications and thickenings seen en face. *B,* Lateral view shows these thickenings much more clearly in profile (upper arrows) anteriorly and posteriorly. The most distinctive finding in asbestos exposure, diaphragmatic calcification, is also seen on the lateral view (*B,* lowest arrow).

EFFUSION

Any sort of fluid may accumulate in the pleural space. This includes water, blood, pus and chyle (Figs. 12–3 and 12–4). A lateral decubitus view with the involved side down will confirm the mobile nature of a pleural collection and allow approximate quantitation (Fig. 1–7). With correct positioning (slightly Trendelenburg), as few as 5 ml. of fluid may be seen on a lateral decubitus film. Several hundred milliliters may hide in the costophrenic angle with the patient erect. Some patients accumulate large amounts of fluid between their lung base and hemidiaphragm with little or no blunting of the lateral or posterior costophrenic angles. This subpulmonic pleural collection mimics an elevated hemidiaphragm. An important hint to a subpulmonic effusion is a shift in the apparent highest portion of the dome of the diaphragm towards the lateral chest wall (Fig. 12–4). Pleural fluid can loculate in fissures ("fluid pseudotumor") or elsewhere in the pleural space. Presumably adhesions or anatomic variants such as incomplete fissures are the cause (Figs. 12–5 and 12–6).

Pleural effusion occurs with congestive heart failure, obstruction of the great veins, fluid and electrolyte imbalance (as with hepatic or renal disease), infection, pulmonary embolism, neoplasm, collagen disease (particularly rheumatoid disease and systemic lupus erythematosus), trauma (check for associated rib fracture and pneumothorax), disruption of the thoracic duct and iatrogenic causes, particularly a malpositioned CVP line (in this case, the collection may be extra- or intrapleural).

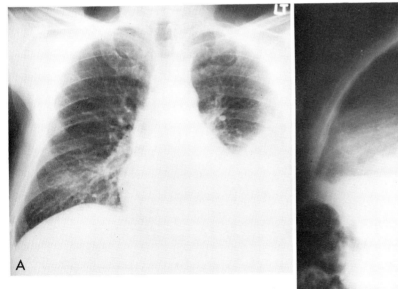

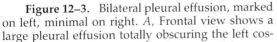

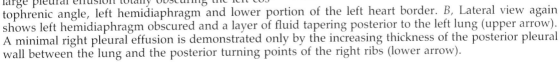

Figure 12–3. Bilateral pleural effusion, marked on left, minimal on right. *A,* Frontal view shows a large pleural effusion totally obscuring the left costophrenic angle, left hemidiaphragm and lower portion of the left heart border. *B,* Lateral view again shows left hemidiaphragm obscured and a layer of fluid tapering posterior to the left lung (upper arrow). A minimal right pleural effusion is demonstrated only by the increasing thickness of the posterior pleural wall between the lung and the posterior turning points of the right ribs (lower arrow).

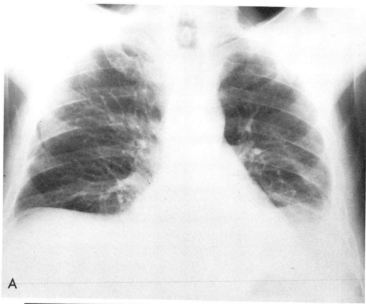

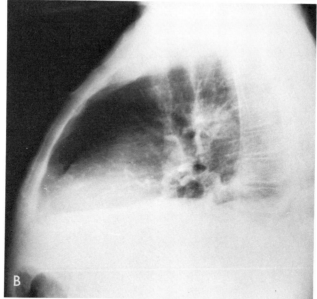

Figure 12–4. Pleural effusions, bilateral, with right subpulmonic. Frontal view (*A*) shows the left hemidiaphragm and costophrenic angle obscured by a pleural effusion, which also obscures the left hemidiaphragm on the lateral view (*B*). A subpulmonic effusion on the right is demonstrable only by the lateral location of the apparent dome on the frontal view (*A*). A right lateral decubitus view (Fig. 1–7) would be necessary to prove the existence of the right pleural effusion.

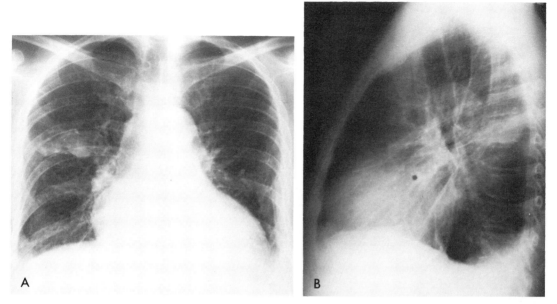

Figure 12–5. Bilateral pleural effusions with loculated effusion, right major fissure. *A,* Frontal view shows blunting of both costophrenic angles and widening of both pleural stripes (left greater than right) inferiorly. A mass density appears present in the right midlung field. *B,* Lateral view shows posterior blunting of both costophrenic angles and also demonstrates the mass to be in the location of the major fissure with the typical fusiform (fattest in the middle) shape of fluid within the fissure.

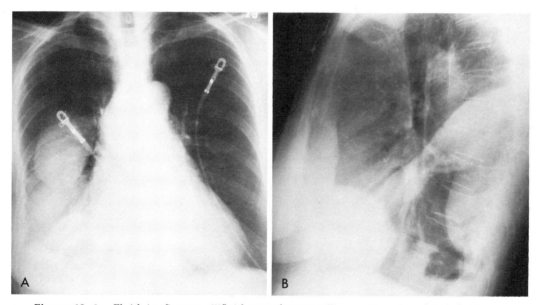

Figure 12–6. Fluid in fissures ("fluid pseudotumors"), massive. Loculated fluid appears masslike on the frontal view (*A*) but is more fusiform on the lateral view (*B*). The upper density on the lateral view represents fluid in the right major fissure, and a loculated posterior effusion is present just beneath it. Costophrenic angle blunting is also evident on the lateral view (*B*).

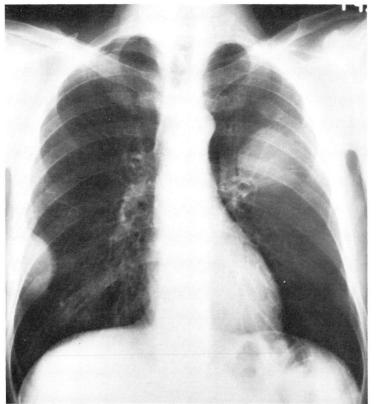

Figure 12–7. Pleural metastases. This young man with a renal carcinoma has bilateral masses on his frontal chest film. The mass in the periphery of the right lung field tapers toward the chest wall in a manner typical of pleural, rather than parenchymal, masses. The mass in the left upper lung field could be either parenchymal or pleural, but suggestions that this mass is pleural include the presence of sharp borders in all directions except laterally and an ill-defined lateral border with tapering toward the pleura. A lateral film confirmed this impression.

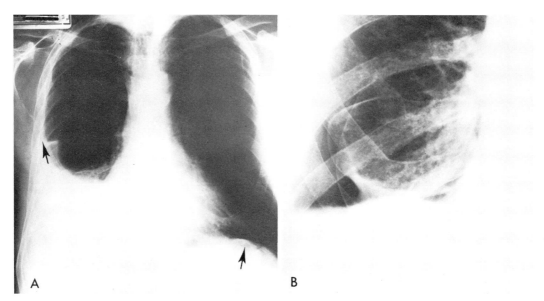

A   B

Figure 12–8. Malignant pleural mesothelioma, localized. The initial frontal view of this asbestos-exposed plumber shows a large right pleural effusion tapering into the lateral portion of the right minor fissure (right arrow). Typical asbestos calcification is seen in the left hemidiaphragm (left arrow). A closeup film (*B*) was obtained following a traumatic thoracentesis resulting in a pneumothorax. Localized thickening of the inferior pleural surface is evident because it is surrounded by the air in the pleural space just above the remaining fluid.

NEOPLASMS

Pleural neoplasms are most commonly due to metastatic disease, especially direct extension from adjacent lung or breast cancer (Fig. 12–7). Malignant mesothelioma is an uncommon primary neoplasm almost always associated with previous asbestos exposure. Radiographic findings can include a thick pleural peel (diffuse pleural thickening), multiple pleural masses and a large pleural effusion (Fig. 12–8).

Benign neoplasms of the pleura include mesothelioma, lipoma (Fig. 12–1) and any other form of mesenchymal tumor.

PNEUMOTHORAX

Pneumothorax can occur spontaneously after cough or straining (Fig. 12–9). This is often associated with an underlying parenchymal abnormality, particularly blebs (Fig. 12–10). Penetrating or blunt trauma also causes a pneumothorax. Necrosis of subpleural lung by infection leads to a bronchopleural fistula and either loculated or free pneumothorax. Extension of air from a pneumomediastinum, a perforated esophagus or trachea can also cause pneumothorax.

If the pathway of air into the pleural space has a ball valve in which air continues to enter the pleural space but cannot escape, the pneumothorax may be under tension (Fig. 12–11). This can be life threatening, since the function of the involved lung is compromised, the mediastinum shifts and the uninvolved lung also cannot function normally. A bilateral pneumothorax presents a similar threat to life.

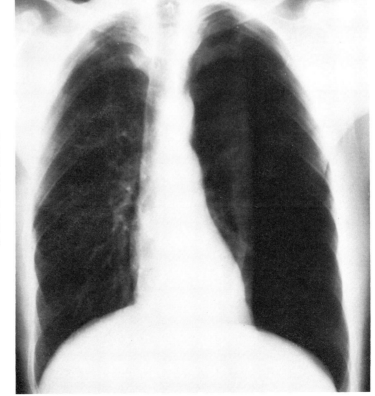

Figure 12–9. Spontaneous pneumothorax. This young man complained of left-sided chest pain but had no history of lung or pleural disease. The frontal film shows a large left pneumothorax with some hyperexpansion of the left hemithorax, indicating mild tension and requiring immediate placement of a chest tube.

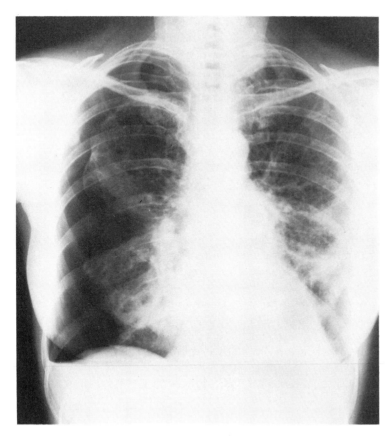

Figure 12–10. Pneumothorax with pleural effusion secondary to chronic (cystic) sarcoid. This middle-aged lady had known pleural and parenchymal lung disease secondary to sarcoid (see Chapter 15). This frontal view shows a large right hydropneumothorax with an air fluid level near the right hemidiaphragm secondary to a small right pleural effusion. Diffuse interstitial parenchymal disease is evident bilaterally.

Often a fluid level is associated with a pneumothorax. In the spontaneous variety this is usually a small amount of blood. The nature of the fluid in other situations depends on the underlying cause of the pneumothorax.

CALCIFICATION

Extensive, irregular visceral pleural calcification, usually unilateral, frequently is due to a previous empyema, often tuberculous. Previous hemothorax can also cause this. Multiple small, irregular calcifications of the parietal pleura are typical of asbestos exposure (Fig. 12–2). Other complications of asbestos exposure such as bronchogenic carcinoma, malignant mesothelioma, and pulmonary fibrosis ("asbestosis") may or may not be present.

EXTRAPLEURAL ABNORMALITIES

Extrapleural densities impinging on the lung are difficult to distinguish from pleural disease. Extrapleural fat or fluid collections maintain their configuration or position with changes in patient position. Extrapleural masses frequently have associated adjacent bone abnormalities as a clue (Fig. 12–12). Hematoma, healed rib fracture, and metastases are common examples. Local views in different projections are often necessary to determine the location and nature of these shadows.

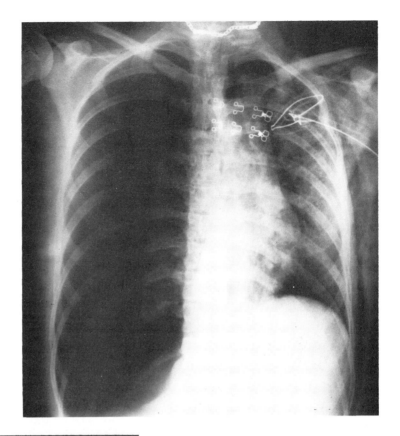

Figure 12–11. Tension pneumothorax, severe, secondary to trauma. This young patient, involved in an auto accident, shows massive inversion of the right hemidiaphragm and displacement of the mediastinum towards the left as the result of a large right tension pneumothorax requiring immediate treatment. Marked subcutaneous emphysema is also noted in the soft tissues on the left. The metallic objects on the left are underneath the patient.

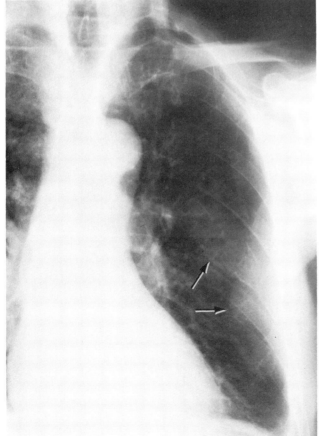

Figure 12–12. Extrapleural mass secondary to metastatic disease. A large pleural mass (lower arrow) appears to taper towards the chest wall at both its upper and lower ends. The seventh posterior rib, adjacent to the mass (upper arrow), is markedly expansile and lytic. Without the abnormal rib, the mass could be either pleural or extrapleural, but the rib abnormality favors an extrapleural mass indenting the lung and continuous with the abnormal rib.

CHAPTER 13

LUNG CANCER

Lung cancer is the most common malignancy (after skin cancer) in the United States. The best available data suggest that early diagnosis increases survival, which currently is still under 10 per cent five years after diagnosis. Unfortunately this highly malignant group of cancers is still increasing in frequency.

Findings on the standard chest roentgenogram are often the first suggestion or major clue that a patient has lung cancer, as symptoms are usually mild and nonspecific and are often attributed to chronic obstructive disease in smokers.

RADIOGRAPHIC FINDINGS

The following radiographic findings may be seen individually or in combination:

1. mass or nodule (Fig. 13–1).
2. enlarged, deformed, dense hilum or mediastinum (Fig. 13–2).
3. segmental, lobar or total lung atelectasis (Fig. 13–3).
4. segmental or lobar consolidation (particularly if this does not resolve or resolves incompletely).
5. a cavity, particularly one with a thick, irregular, nodular wall.
6. a persistent, growing area of consolidation (often alveolar cell cancer) (Fig. 13–4).
7. poorly defined parenchymal density, particularly in the lung apex.
8. bone destruction, which can be from metastatic disease or direct invasion of the chest wall. The latter is most typically seen in Pancoast tumors of the lung apex.
9. septal lines. These can be due to tumor spread or venous and lymphatic obstruction.
10. pleural effusion. This is most often due to tumor involvement of the pleura but may be secondary to inflammatory disease or venous or lymphatic obstruction.
11. a narrowed trachea or bronchus. A protuberant mass or extrinsic compression can cause this.
12. an elevated hemidiaphragm. Atelectasis or paralysis of a phrenic nerve can be the etiology.
13. hyperinflation of a lobe or segment due to a ball valve mechanism in the bronchus (rare).

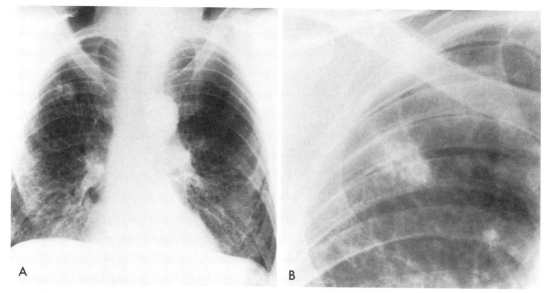

Figure 13–1. Adenocarcinoma, right upper lobe. Frontal film *(A)* and close-up of the right upper lung field *(B)* show a very poorly defined mass in the periphery. As is typical of peripheral adenocarcinomas, this mass was discovered on a routine film and caused no symptoms (AFIP negative #67–5185).

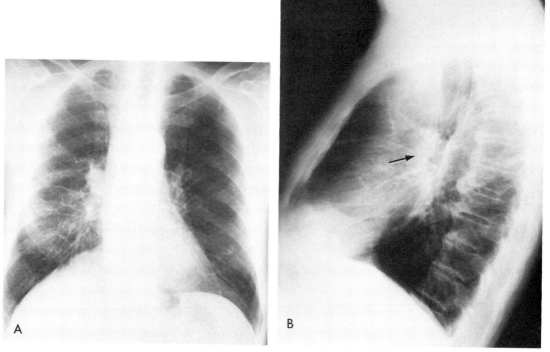

Figure 13–2. Squamous bronchogenic carcinoma, right hilum. A mass is evident on the frontal view *(A)* in the superior portion of the right hilum. The mass is less distinct on the lateral view *(B)* but is seen (arrow) just above the right pulmonary artery and anterior to the right mainstem bronchus.

Figure 13–3. Squamous carcinoma, left mainstem bronchus, with total atelectasis of left lung. The homogeneous opacification of the left lung and marked deviation of the mediastinum towards the left suggest total left lung atelectasis. The left mainstem bronchus is abruptly cut off where it is obstructed (arrow). There is marked compensatory hypertrophy of the right lung. The findings on this film could also be consistent with a ball valve mechanism obstructing the right mainstem bronchus were it not for the sharp cutoff of the left mainstem bronchus.

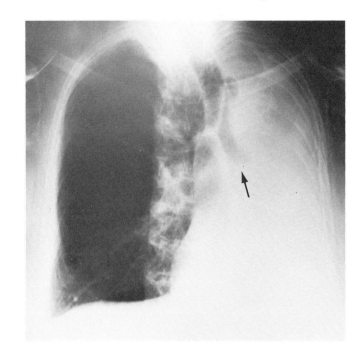

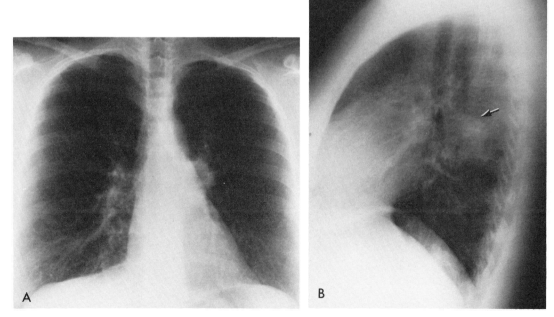

Figure 13–4. Broncho-alveolar cell carcinoma, superior segment of left lower lobe. On the frontal view (A) a mass appears present in the left hilum. The lateral view (B) shows that the density is in fact a poorly defined infiltrate in the superior segment of the left lower lobe (arrow) significantly posterior to the hilum. The infiltrate resembles a pneumonia, but its persisting presence in the absence of symptoms of pneumonia suggested the correct diagnosis (which was confirmed surgically).

14. hyperlucency of a segment, lobe or lung due to decreased vascular supply. This is usually difficult to appreciate on the plain films but is frequently demonstrated by perfusion lung scan.
15. a bronchocele. A slowly progressive neoplasm (either a carcinoma or adenoma) may occlude a bronchus, which dilates and fills with mucus distal to the obstruction.
16. dilatation of the superior vena cava and/or azygos veins due to mediastinal tumor spread.

ADDITIONAL RADIOGRAPHIC EVALUATION

In any individual case, further radiographic evaluation may be appropriate.

1. **Oblique films** at various degrees can confirm the presence of an abnormality and localize it. Standard tomograms in the AP, lateral or oblique projection can confirm or localize a lesion as well as show its relationship to adjacent structures (bones, hilum, mediastinum, diaphragm, fissures).
2. **Computerized tomography** is more sensitive than conventional methods for detection of tiny lung nodules. It is also the best noninvasive way of documenting direct invasion of adjacent structures and mediastinal extension of malignancy (Figs. 13–5 and 13–6).
3. **Fluoroscopy** demonstrates diaphragmatic paralysis, is very useful in localizing small lesions, and is the easiest technique to use to verify the presence or absence of calcification.
4. **Ventilation and perfusion lung scans** show the physiology of areas affected by the neoplasm and also assess the relative function of other areas of the lung. This may be particularly helpful in determining operability.
5. **Other pertinent examinations** should be requested when appropriate because of historical, physical and laboratory findings. These include plain films, computerized tomographic studies (particularly of the brain) and radio-isotopic bone and liver scans. Current information suggests that none of these studies should be routine in the evaluation of all lung cancers, but there is debate over this point.

CYTOLOGIC EXAMINATION

The diagnosis of lung cancer suggested by radiographic findings must be confirmed cytologically or pathologically. Methods for diagnosis, in order of increasing morbidity, are:

a. sputum cytologic analysis
b. bronchoscopic biopsy and washings
c. biopsy of a distant metastasis
d. needle aspiration of a lung, hilar or mediastinal abnormality
e. mediastinoscopic biopsy
f. thoracostomy with biopsy
g. thoracotomy with biopsy and, if appropriate, resection

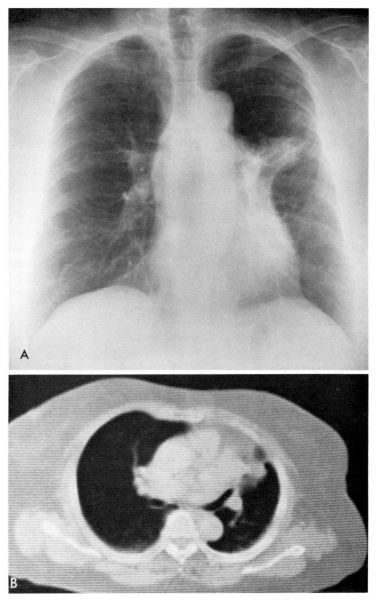

Figure 13–5. Carcinoma, poorly differentiated, involving mediastinum and chest wall by direct extension. *A,* Frontal chest film
shows partial obstruction of the left upper lobe with a mass visible in
the left hilar region. *B,* One view from a computerized tomogram
shows continuity of soft tissue density from anterior chest wall into
the mediastinum, indicating involvement of both of these areas as well
as the intervening lung.

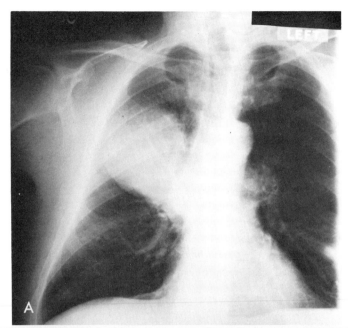

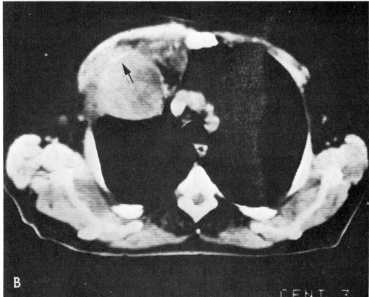

Figure 13–6. Poorly differentiated squamous carcinoma, right upper lobe, with extension to chest wall. *A,* A large homogeneous mass in the right upper lobe with distortion of the right hilum is visible on the frontal chest film. *B,* A view from the computerized tomogram shows direct extension of the mass into the right anterior chest wall with marked expansion of the soft tissues (compared with those on the left side) and rib destruction (small remnant indicated by arrow).

SURGERY

Carcinoma of the lung must also be staged for appropriate therapy. Surgical removal currently offers the best chance for long-term cure but is often not possible. Surgery should not be performed if:

1. other medical conditions make it dangerous (often there is severe chronic obstructive lung disease or cardiac disease).
2. a distant metastasis is present.
3. contralateral lung metastasis is documented.
4. the mediastinum is involved by direct extension or nodal metastasis. Sometimes this is suggested by involvement of the recurrent laryngeal or phrenic nerve.
5. a malignant pleural effusion is present.
6. direct invasion of the chest wall is noted. All these patients have local or referred pain. Some surgical cures have been effected in these patients, particularly those with Pancoast tumors treated first with radiation. The decision for surgery in such a patient is a complicated one depending on the patient's condition and available surgical expertise.

The order of diagnostic and staging procedures depends upon findings in the individual patient, available equipment and professional skills. Although precise data are unavailable, probably 20 to 50 per cent of patients with an abnormal chest roentgenogram due to lung cancer are not diagnosed as early as possible. Patients who have changes reported that could be due to lung cancer are not diagnosed because they fail to return to their physician; the radiographic report is not received by the referring physician; or the referring physician chooses to ignore abnormalities reported. Findings on the films can also be misinterpreted as being of no significance or may simply not be observed. Results can be improved by double reading, knowledge of typical radiographic patterns of lung cancer and careful comparison with previous studies.

COMMON CELL TYPES OF LUNG CANCER

Epidermoid (squamous cell) cancer typically presents as a central mass (Fig. 13–2). These central lesions are often easily diagnosed by sputum cytology or bronchoscopy. A normal chest roentgenogram with positive sputum cytology for epidermoid cancer should lead to a careful workup that includes fiberoptic bronchoscopy and evaluation for head and neck or esophageal origin. Careful evaluation of these areas will sometimes discover an early primary malignancy.

Adenocarcinoma often presents as a shaggy or stellate peripheral nodule (Fig. 13–1). Unfortunately, if the lesion is poorly differentiated, even the discovery at the stage of a small asymptomatic peripheral nodule does not guarantee cure, since early metastases are the rule.

Oat cell cancer is rarely cured by any method, since it has almost always spread hematogenously by the time of discovery. Most oncologists recommend that surgery not be performed in patients with proven oat cell cancer. This form of malignancy is sensitive to radiation and/or chemotherapy with occasional long-term survival and frequent palliation of symptoms. The chest radiograph often shows extensive hilar and mediastinal lymph node involvement (Fig. 13–7).

Alveolar cell carcinoma is less common than the other varieties. It may present with any radiographic findings but typically is a slowly growing, poorly defined peripheral infiltrate or mass that is mistaken for pneumonia or scarring (Fig. 13–4). At some time in the course of the disease multiple areas of one or both lungs can be involved with consolidation or alveolar-type nodules.

Bronchial adenoma is also an uncommon form of lung neoplasm, and it is classified as a very low-grade carcinoma. It is usually manifest as a well-circumscribed hilar or perihilar mass (Fig. 13–8). Approximately 85 per cent of bronchial adenomas are carcinoids. Unless adequate excision is done, these tumors recur locally. Rarely, direct extension to vital structures or distant spread occurs before initial diagnosis and surgery. Unlike the other forms of lung cancer, which principally affect men of 50 to 80 years, this neoplasm is more common in young adults.

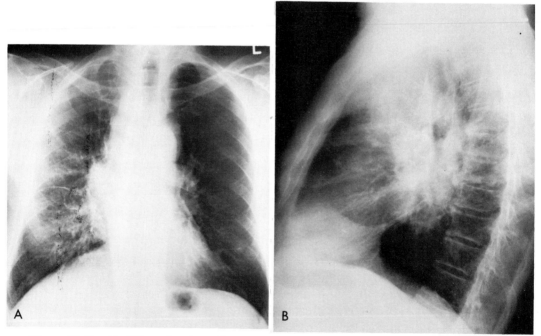

Figure 13–7. Undifferentiated small cell (oat cell) carcinoma, right hilum and mediastinum. Massive, irregular enlargement of the right hilum is evident on both frontal *(A)* and lateral *(B)* views. The right paratracheal area on the frontal view is also markedly widened, indicating severe paratracheal lymphadenopathy. Lymphangitic spread in the right lung is shown by the marked thickening of the vascular markings on the frontal view.

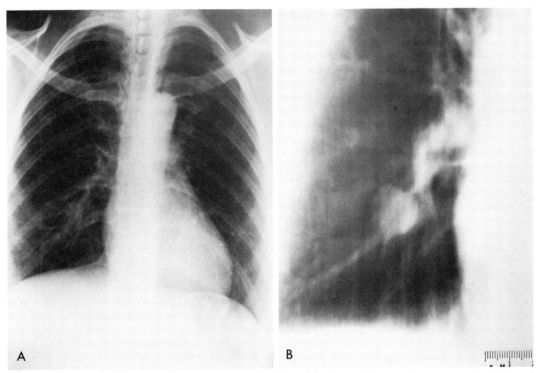

Figure 13–8. Bronchial adenoma, carcinoid type, right lower lobe. *A,* The frontal chest film of this asymptomatic young lady shows an extremely subtle mass in the right lower lung field medially. A frontal tomogram *(B)* clearly shows the well-circumscribed and round appearance of a bronchial adenoma.

CHAPTER 14

METASTASES AND LYMPHOMAS

METASTASES

Metastatic disease may present as mediastinal or hilar lymphadenopathy or may cause pulmonary abnormalities. The appearance of pulmonary metastases depends upon the mode of spread *through* the lung rather than *to* the lung. Thus, a carcinoma that spreads lymphogenously throughout the body causing diffuse lymphadenopathy may also cause hematogenous metastases in the lungs and vice versa.

Hematogenous metastatic spread in the lung is generally characterized by small interstitial nodules (Fig. 14–1) that may grow rapidly and become more hazy, especially if they cause hemorrhage. The nodules are more often subpleural and basilar because of the prevalence of small vessels and increased blood flow in these regions. An overpenetrated view of the lower lung fields is often very helpful in seeing such nodules in the portion of the lower lobes behind the diaphragms. Common causes of hematogenous metastatic disease include sarcomas, melanomas, trophoblastic malignancies, thyroid carcinomas, carcinoids, adenocarcinomas of breast, colon or pancreas and squamous carcinomas, especially from the head and the neck region. However, virtually any malignancy may cause these nodules.

Lymphogenous metastatic disease in the lungs appears as diffuse interstitial infiltration most marked in the lower lung fields, especially near the hila (Fig. 14–2). Nodularity may be present but is much more ill-defined than in hematogenous metastatic disease and generally is distributed with the bronchovascular structures (Fig. 14–3). The appearance of lymphogenous spread very much resembles interstitial pulmonary edema except for the absence of other signs of congestion, especially enlargement of upper lobe vessels that is usually seen in interstitial edema (see Chapter 18). Common causes include carcinomas of breast, stomach, lung and lower GU tract, including the prostate.

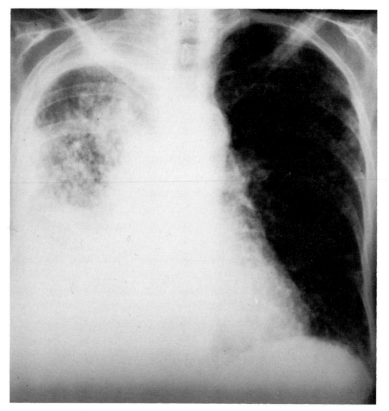

Figure 14–1. Hematogenous metastatic disease secondary to renal cell carcinoma. Multiple small nodules are present in both lung fields. They are slightly confluent and less well defined in areas of greatest profusion, such as in the periphery of the left upper lung field. Marked right pleural thickening, a large right pleural effusion and mediastinal widening due to lymphadenopathy are also present.

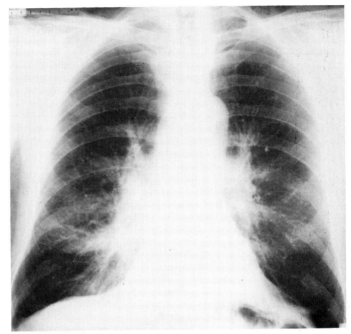

Figure 14–2. Lymphogenous metastatic disease secondary to adenocarcinoma of the stomach. A reticular interstitial pattern is seen, especially in the medial portion of the lower lung fields. The hila are diffusely enlarged bilaterally. This appearance should be contrasted with that of congestive failure (Chapter 18).

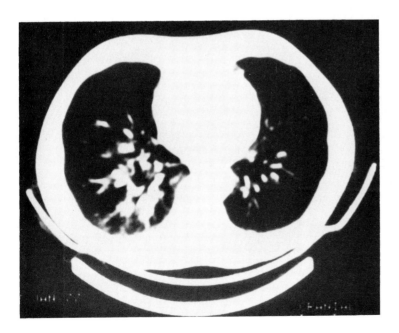

Figure 14–3. Lymphogenous metastatic disease from adenocarcinoma of unknown origin. This CT at the level of the pulmonary veins shows marked nodular dilatation of the bronchovascular markings in the right lower lung field, especially the right lower lobe. The vessels in the left lower lung field also show minimal nodularity.

LYMPHOMAS

All lymphomas cause enlarged lymph nodes in hila and mediastinum more often than any other chest film abnormalities. The lymph node enlargement may be localized or diffuse and is especially diffuse in highly malignant lymphomas (Fig. 14–4).

Hodgkin's disease invades the lung in late, severe cases (Stage IV) (Fig. 14–5). Nodules and small masses are usually present and the masses often cavitate (Fig. 14–6). An appearance resembling lymphogenous metastatic disease may occur but is usually more nodular.

Non-Hodgkin's lymphomas and, rarely, Hodgkin's lymphomas, may originate in the lung as consolidative infiltrates, often with an air bronchogram resembling pneumonia or alveolar cell bronchogenic carcinoma (Fig. 2–4). Lymphadenopathy may be absent. Open biopsy is usually necessary for diagnosis of this lesion, as benign lymphoid infiltrates (pseudolymphoma and lymphocytic interstitial pneumonitis) may be radiologically identical to pulmonary lymphoma.

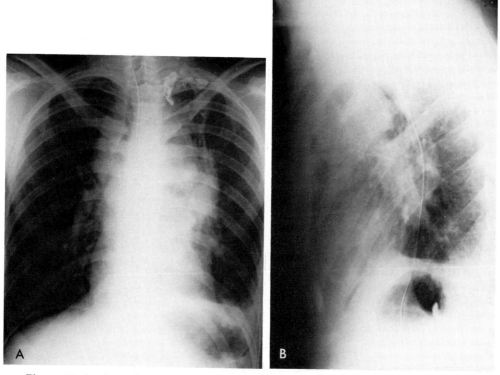

Figure 14–4. Lymphoma, undifferentiated. *A,* Frontal view. *B,* Lateral view. Massive mediastinal lymphadenopathy is demonstrated by marked widening of the mediastinum, marked thickening of the right paratracheal region, splaying of the carina, complete loss of ability to see the descending aorta and aortic knob and by lateral displacement and enlargement of the left hilum. This patient also has a pneumoperitoneum visible beneath the right hemidiaphragm and has residual contrast in the left apex from a lymphangiogram. A nasogastric tube is also visible, and there is a left pleural effusion.

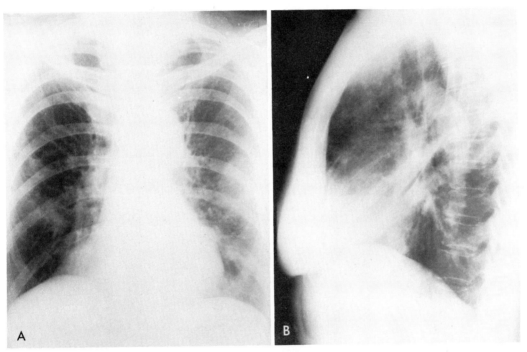

Figure 14–5. Hodgkin's disease, Stage IV. Multiple ill-defined nodules and infiltrates are present in both lung fields. Diffuse mediastinal widening, obscuring the aortic knob on the frontal view *(A)*, and right hilar enlargement are also visible on both frontal and lateral *(B)* views.

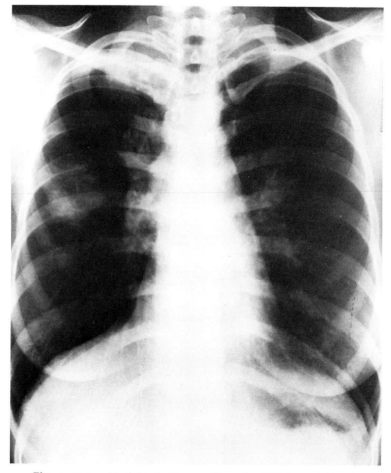

Figure 14–6. Hodgkin's disease, Stage IV. This frontal film shows a large cavitary mass in the center of the right upper lung field. Diffuse infiltration is also present around the right hilum and there is nodular widening of the mediastinum.

CHAPTER 15

PULMONARY EMBOLISM

Pulmonary embolism is a common problem, particularly in hospitalized or immobilized patients and in those with cardiac disease or malignancy or in those on oral contraceptives.

The majority of patients with pulmonary embolism have a normal chest roentgenogram. Most of the others have one or more nonspecific findings, including linear atelectasis, pleural effusion, elevation of a hemidiaphragm and patchy consolidation. Uncommonly, the chest film findings strongly suggest embolic disease. These more specific findings include:

1. dense, peripheral consolidation, particularly if based on a pleural surface(s) (Fig. 15–1). If the medial surface is convex, this is referred to as a Hampton's hump.
2. an enlarged, amputated major pulmonary artery.
3. one or more areas of decreased vasculature not due to bullae or emphysema. This sign (Westermark's sign) is usually difficult to see (Fig. 15–2).

PERFUSION SCAN

If pulmonary embolism is suspected, a perfusion scan should be performed (Fig. 15–3A).

If the perfusion (Q) scan is:

1. normal—the workup should stop. The patient does not have a pulmonary embolism.
2. abnormal only in areas of chest film abnormality—this is a nonspecific combination that will not be resolved by a ventilation scan.
3. abnormal in areas that are normal on the chest film—a ventilation scan should be performed.

VENTILATION SCAN

If the ventilation scan (Fig. 15–3B) is abnormal (showing obstruction to inflow or air trapping) in areas corresponding to the abnormalities on the perfusion scan, pulmonary embolism is unlikely.

If the ventilation scan is normal in areas that are abnormal on the perfusion scan, very small mismatched areas are nonspecific; segmental or larger mismatched areas are usually due to pulmonary embolism.

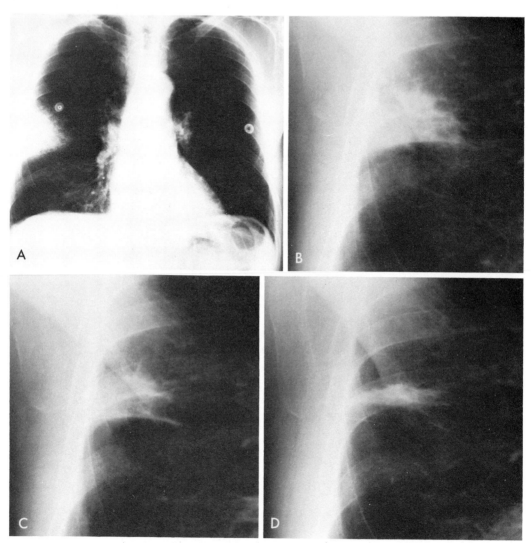

Figure 15–1. Pulmonary embolism and infarction with infiltrate. *A,* Initial frontal film shows a pleural-based triangular infiltrate in the right mid lung field with a convex inner border facing towards the hilum (Hampton's hump). *B,* Closeup view of the right mid lung field made four days later shows decreased size of infiltrate and clear evidence that infiltrate is segmental in the anterior segment of the right upper lobe. The sharp lower border of the infiltrate is the minor fissure. *C,* Six days later, the lesion is still smaller but remains as dense as previously. The tendency of infarcts to become smaller without loss of density is often referred to as the "melting sign." It is an unreliable sign in differentiating pneumonia from infarction during the healing phase. *D,* Two weeks later, the lesion resembles a linear scar as it continues to contract or "melt."

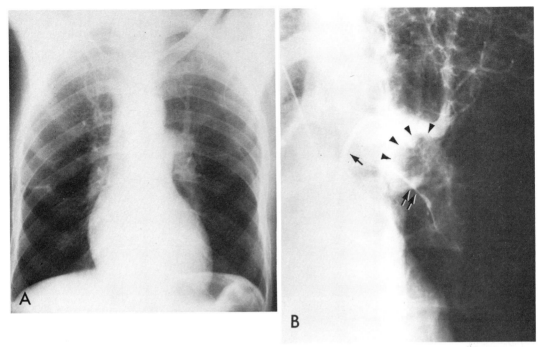

Figure 15–2. Pulmonary embolism, left pulmonary artery. *A,* Frontal chest film shows extremely subtle decrease in vascular shadows in the left mid and lower lung fields (Westermark's sign). The decreased vascularity is only visible by careful comparison of left and right lung fields. The left pulmonary artery appears prominent but not definitely abnormal. *B,* Closeup view of left pulmonary artery during arteriogram shows catheter (arrow) emerging from right ventricular outflow tract with tip in left pulmonary artery. An artery supplying the apex of the left upper lobe is filled. No significant flow to the remainder of the left lung is seen, except for a thin rim of contrast (double arrow) in the inferior portion of the left pulmonary arterty beneath the large thrombus (arrowheads).

The result of the V/Q scan and chest roentgenogram may, therefore, be nondiagnostic, particularly in a patient with congestive heart failure or chronic obstructive lung disease. The decision for anticoagulant therapy must then be based on clinical criteria or a pulmonary angiogram should be performed (Fig. 15–3C).

ANGIOGRAPHY

Pulmonary angiography (Figs. 15–2 and 15–3) is the most specific test for pulmonary embolism. If performed correctly, both false positive and false negative results are rare. Expense, patient discomfort and possible morbidity and mortality all make referring physicians hesitant to order this examination. Morbidity and mortality are small only if the person performing the examination is experienced.

Newer generation CT equipment can show clot in the larger pulmonary arteries after intravenous contrast injection. With software improvement and experience, this technique may become more valuable in the management of pulmonary embolism.

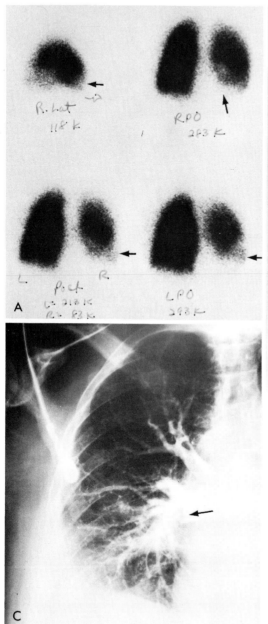

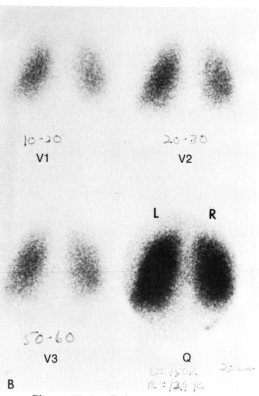

Figure 15–3. Pulmonary embolism, right lower lobe. *A,* Four views from perfusion (Q) scan show a segmental defect in the postero-lateral portion of the right lower lobe (arrows). The right lung also shows diffuse diminished perfusion compared with the normal left lung. *B,* Three views from the "washout" phase of the ventilation (V) scan show minimal decreased ventilation to the entire right lung (the right lung is on your right since this is a posterior view and displayed, by convention, the same way the view is obtained). No defect corresponds to the segmental defect on the Q scan. *C,* Frontal view of pulmonary angiogram shows a clot in the lower portion of the right pulmonary artery (arrow). The peripheral filling in the lower lung field is mostly middle lobe rather than lower lobe.

CHAPTER 16

GRANULOMATOUS DISEASE

Granulomatous inflammation is a common cause of chest film abnormalities involving the pulmonary parenchyma, hila, pleura and mediastinum. The parenchymal disease represents a localized response (usually multifocal) to an infection or other insult and is, therefore, manifest in most cases as nodules or masses. Pleural involvement consists of diffuse or multinodular inflammation. The propensity for marked lymph node enlargement by granulomatous inflammation often diffusely enlarges lymph nodes in hila and the mediastinum.

Both infectious and noninfectious insults may stimulate the granulomatous reaction. Common infectious granulomatous diseases include tuberculosis, atypical mycobacterial infection, histoplasmosis, coccidioidomycosis, blastomycosis, cryptococcosis and actinomycosis. Despite individual differences among the diseases caused by these organisms, a markedly similar pattern of infection and clinical and radiographic abnormalities are found. The most common noninfectious granulomatous disease is sarcoid, but there are many others, including silicosis, berylliosis and Wegener's granulomatosis.

DISEASE FORMS

Forms of infectious granulomatous disease include:

1. **Primary Infection.** Inhalation of organisms leads to the development of pneumonia (Figs. 16–1 and 16–2). Draining lymph nodes become involved but often fail to filter out all of the organisms. The organisms that escape the nodes pass into the thoracic duct and then the blood. Dissemination of these organisms to the lung and other organs occurs. This stage of granulomatous infection is usually asymptomatic, but the pneumonia, lymphadenopathy or disseminated disease may produce clinically apparent illness.

2. **Pleural Effusion.** In some patients the primary infection extends to the pleura and a pleural effusion develops. This is frequently asymptomatic, and examination of pleural fluid is usually not diagnostic. A pleural effusion in a young adult with a positive tuberculin skin test is due to tuberculosis unless proven otherwise.

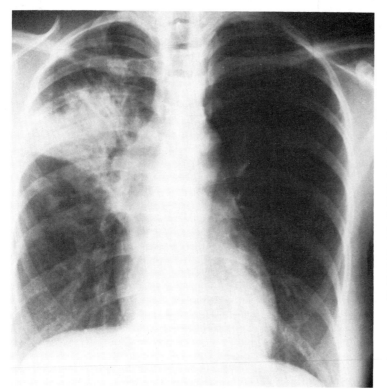

Figure 16–1. Granulomatous pneumonia, primary pulmonary tuberculosis. Alveolar
consolidation is present in the
right upper lung field, especially
the anterior segment just above
the minor fissure. Marked right
hilar lymphadenopathy is present, enlarging the right hilum
and making it appear nodular.
The high position of the minor
fissure suggests that right upper
lobe volume loss is being caused
by lymph nodes obstructing the
right upper lobe bronchus.

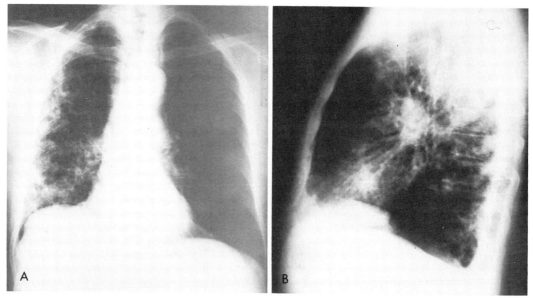

Figure 16–2. Granulomatous pneumonia, diffuse, probably histoplasmosis. Frontal *(A)* and
lateral *(B)* views show a diffuse pneumonic process involving the periphery of the right lung field
with minimal right volume loss. The character of the infiltrate is mixed consolidative and interstitial,
a common finding in granulomatous pneumonias. No significant lymphadenopathy is seen, and
the appearance in this case is far less specific than the combination of consolidation and lymph
node enlargement seen in Figure 16–1.

3. Reactivation (Secondary or Cavitary) Disease. The initial dissemination of organisms or re-exposure to exogenous organisms may lead to this form of granulomatous infection, which is most common in the apical and posterior segments of the upper lobes (Fig. 16–3). Heavy exposure, malnutrition (including that caused by diabetes, alcoholism, drug abuse, GI surgery, or poverty) and immunosuppression predispose to secondary disease. This form of disease often has cavitation, fibrosis and upper lobe volume loss on the films. The incidence and predisposition to chronic cavitary disease vary markedly among the granulomatous infections. Histoplasmosis, for example, only manifests as chronic cavitary disease in individuals with underlying chronic obstructive pulmonary disease.

4. Extrapulmonary Involvement. Any organ system may be infected from the hematogenous dissemination. Other pathways of infection are rare.

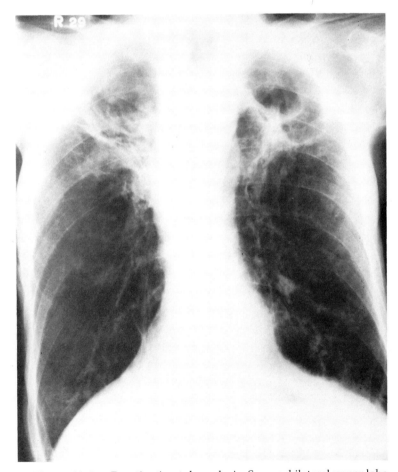

Figure 16–3. Reactivation tuberculosis. Severe, bilateral upper lobe scarring and cyst formation are present. Hazy infiltrates and nodules are present throughout the lungs, especially adjacent to the cystic regions, and many hazy nodules are present in the left lung. The mediastinum is widened superiorly. Emphysema is also present. Activity is difficult to judge with this appearance, but the presence of hazy densities in addition to the sharp, dense linear scars favors present activity.

5. Symptomatic Disseminated Disease. Progressive disseminated disease in the lungs and multiple other organs is life threatening. It may occur after the initial exposure or re-exposure or during the course of active pulmonary infection. Disseminated tuberculosis and most other granulomatous infections are more common in blacks and the immuno-suppressed. A miliary pattern is often present on the chest roentgenogram (Fig. 16–4).

6. Hilar and Mediastinal Lymphadenopathy. This form of the disease is rarely symptomatic, but bronchial, vascular and esophageal compression can occur. Calcification of these nodes is common months to years after the initial infection, especially in TBC and histoplasmosis, but rarely if ever in coccidioidomycosis (Fig. 16–5).

7. Residua of Past Infection. Many chest films have footprints from previous granulomatous infection. These include:

    a. parenchymal nodules that are often partially or completely calcified (Fig. 16–6).

    b. calcified lymph nodes (Fig. 16–6).

    c. upper lobe volume loss, irregular fibrotic shadows and/or calcification.

    d. pleural thickening, adhesion and calcification (Fig. 16–7).

    e. splenic calcifications (nearly always from histoplasmosis).

Classical tuberculosis due to *Mycobacterium tuberculosis* var. *hominis* is an infectious disease passed from person to person. These organisms can

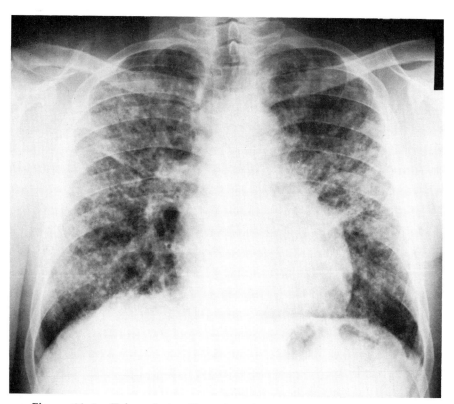

Figure 16–4. Tuberculosis, disseminated. Diffuse, ill-defined nodules are present throughout both lung fields. Areas of alveolar confluence are present, especially in the periphery of both lungs. These findings, or the multiple sharp, tiny nodules of miliary disease (see Chapter 5), are typical of disseminated granulomatous disease.

Table 16–1. EPIDEMIOLOGY OF GRANULOMATOUS DISEASE

Organism	Common Forms of Disease*	U.S. Epidemiology
Mycobacterium	3,2,5,1; 7a,b,c,d	Large cities, jails, immigrants
Atypical Mycobacterium	3, 7c	Group III, esp. Battey: Southeast; Group I (kansasii): South and Midwest
Histoplasma	6,1,5,3; 7a–b,e	Large river valleys, including entire Midwest and Southeast
Coccidioides	1,4,6,7a	Deserts of Southwest and California; as far east as Texas
Blastomyces	1,4	Southeast and Midwest
Cryptococcus	1,4,7a	All United States

*Numbers refer to accompanying list of disease forms, pp. 99–103.

live for a long time in soil or dust. All of the other forms of granulomatous infection are not considered contagious except in rare circumstances. Because of this, isolation of infected individuals is not recommended except with active untreated tuberculosis. All of these other organisms have soil reservoirs that lead to human infection, occasionally in epidemic form. Animal vectors are common in some of the infections, especially histoplasmosis.

Microbiologic techniques are used to determine the activity of an infectious granulomatous disease process and which organism is causing the infection. Any changing radiographic pattern is presumptive evidence of active infection.

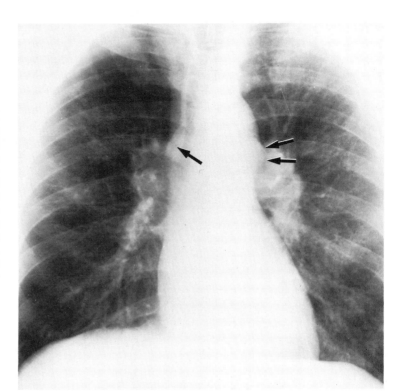

Figure 16–5. Hilar and mediastinal lymphadenopathy, granulomatous. Bilateral hilar enlargement is present, and mediastinal lymphadenopathy is obvious in the right paratracheal (azygous) area (single arrow) and in the aortopulmonary window (double arrow). Hazy infiltrates are seen in both upper lung fields. This appearance is common in both infectious and noninfectious granulomatous disease.

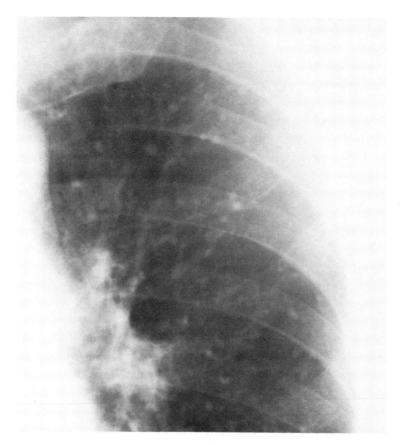

Figure 16–6. Histoplasmosis, multiple calcified nodules and lymph nodes. Multiple calcified nodules are present throughout the left upper lobe in this closeup of that region, and there are multiple hilar calcifications in lymph nodes. Completely calcified nodules, as here, are more common in noninfectious diseases such as silicosis than in infectious diseases such as histoplasmosis, in which only the center of the peripheral nodule usually cavitates.

Figure 16–7. Tuberculosis, healed, postsurgical. A large, dense pleural thickening is present in the left apex with calcification along the remaining pleural surface (arrows). The right lung has been completely collapsed by a thoracoplasty.

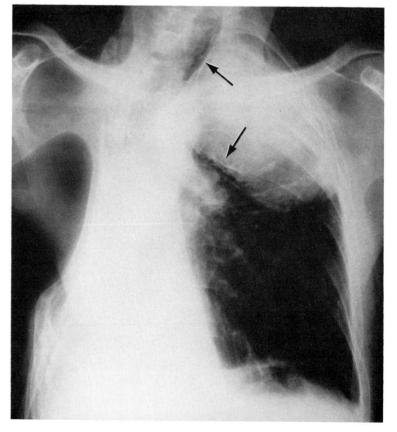

SARCOIDOSIS

Sarcoidosis is a common disease of young adults, especially black women. The cause is unknown. Geographical distribution is striking, with high incidence in the southeastern and eastern United States and in Scandinavia.

Sarcoidosis most commonly involves lymph nodes (Fig. 16–8) and pulmonary interstitium, but any organ may be affected.

Patients with sarcoidosis are often asymptomatic, especially in early disease with only nodal involvement. Nodal and parenchymal lung disease may be extensive, with the radiograph appearing far worse than the symptoms, a strong clue to the diagnosis. Although sarcoidosis is usually self-limited, parenchymal lung involvement may progress to fibrosis (Fig. 16–9). Most pulmonary physicians treat patients who have severely abnormal arterial blood gases or progressive disease with steroids in an attempt to decrease permanent damage.

Symmetrical hilar and mediastinal lymphadenopathy without parenchymal lung disease is the most common radiographic pattern (Fig. 16–8). Parenchymal involvement may coincide with or follow the nodal enlargement.

Common radiographic patterns include reticular, reticulonodular and fluffy coalescent nodule(s). Although pathologically the disease is interstitial, severe involvement may produce alveolar consolidation with fluffy densities and air bronchograms on the radiograph (Fig. 16–10). Pleural effusion and nodal compression with symptoms are uncommon.

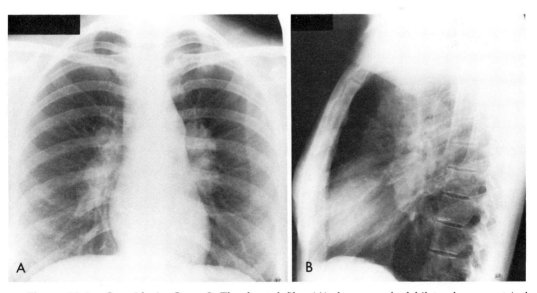

Figure 16–8. Sarcoidosis, Stage I. The frontal film *(A)* shows marked bilateral, symmetrical hilar enlargement due to lymph nodes. The mediastinum, especially the right paratracheal region and aortopulmonary window, also contains enlarged lymph nodes. As is characteristic of sarcoid, the lymph node enlargement is symmetrical and the hila appear to "stick out" from the mediastinum. The lateral film *(B)* shows the marked hilar enlargement as multiple nodules surrounding the pulmonary arteries.

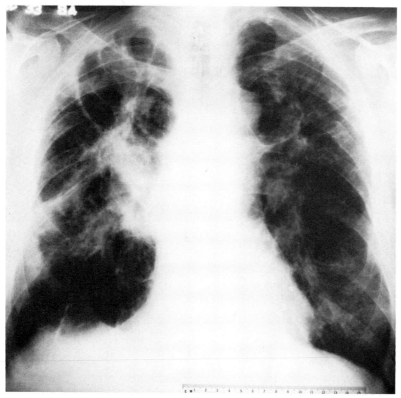

Figure 16–9. Sarcoidosis, Stage III. Marked upper lobe fibro-bullous disease is present. Confluent infiltrations surround the right hilum, and the mediastinum is widened and nodular. The large size of the upper lobe cysts makes sarcoid more likely than other granulomatous diseases in this case.

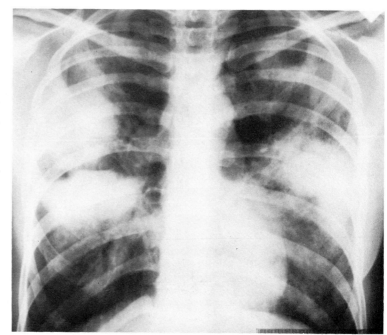

Figure 16–10. Sarcoidosis, Stage II—"alveolar sarcoid." Large areas of consolidation are present in both lung fields, especially in the periphery. Ill-defined infiltration is also present elsewhere and is most obvious at the left base. Lymphadenopathy is not clearly present, as it is common in sarcoid for the lymphadenopathy to decrease while the parenchymal changes are still clearly seen.

INHALATION DISEASES

The airways and pulmonary parenchyma are damaged by a wide variety of inhaled gases, particles and fluids. Typical radiographic manifestations may be present in these conditions.

PNEUMOCONIOSES (INORGANIC DUST)

SILICOSIS

Particles of silica are inhaled during a variety of mining and industrial situations, including coal mining, quarrying, sand blasting and foundry work.

Reaction to the inhaled silica particles leads to the development of an interstitial nodular pattern (Fig. 17–1), which is often more pronounced in the upper lung fields. With progression, volume loss and fibrosis occur. In some patients the small nodular densities coalesce to form irregular masses (conglomerate nodules or progressive massive fibrosis). At this stage of the disease clinical and radiographic progression may continue without further exposure to silica (Fig. 17–2).

Involvement of hilar and mediastinal lymph nodes causes moderate enlargement, often with a characteristic calcified rim (eggshell calcification).

Patients with silicosis are predisposed to develop pulmonary tuberculosis, but silica exposure does not cause an increase in lung cancer incidence.

ASBESTOS DISEASES

Exposure to asbestos fibers is heaviest in asbestos mines, asbestos processing plants, construction using asbestos insulation materials, shipyards and a wide variety of other work environments. However, clinically significant asbestos exposure may occur in the neighborhood of asbestos plants and to family members of asbestos workers. Asbestos usage is increasing, creating a significant public health problem.

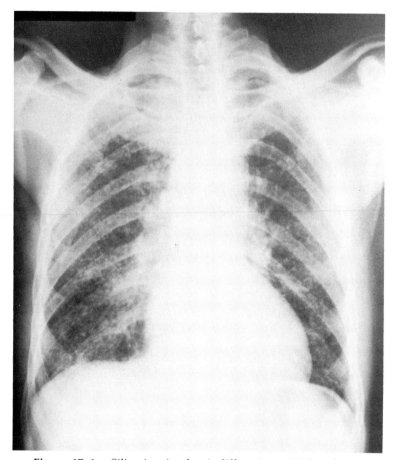

Figure 17–1. Silicosis, simple. A diffuse interstitial nodular (reticulonodular) pattern is present throughout both lung fields. The hila are enlarged bilaterally secondary to lymphadenopathy. This appearance is typical of early silica inhalation, especially in individuals exposed to finely divided particles, such as in sandblasting or glassmaking. The term "simple" refers to nodules smaller than 1 cm. in diameter.

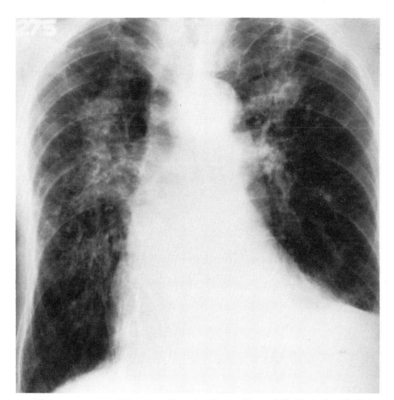

Figure 17–2. Silicosis, chronic "complicated." Ill-defined, hazy densities are present in the medial portion of both upper lung fields (conglomerate nodules or progressive massive fibrosis). Bilateral upper lobe volume loss is present, and some calcification of the nodules, especially in the left hilum, is also visible. Scattered, irregular nodules are present elsewhere, especially in the upper lung fields. The term "complicated" refers to the old belief, never well proven, that such conglomerate lesions (larger than 1 cm. in diameter by definition) involve tuberculosis or some other complication in addition to silica inhalation. The appearance here is identical to that in coal workers' pneumoconiosis, which is a different, and less clinically significant, disease.

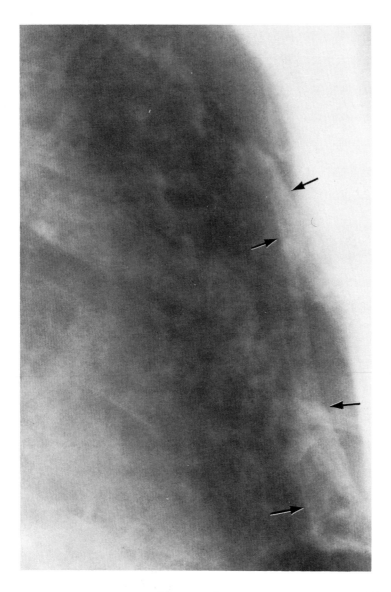

Figure 17–3. Asbestos pleural plaques. A long linear plaque with some calcification is seen in this closeup of the left mid lung field of a patient with a long history of asbestos exposure. Such findings are usually bilateral; when unilateral, old inflammatory disease rather than asbestos exposure is usually the cause.

Heavy asbestos exposure causes diffuse interstitial fibrosis ("asbestosis") which is usually most pronounced at the lung bases (Fig. 4–5). Pulmonary insufficiency may result.

Common pleural abnormalities include small effusions, plaques, and calcifications (Figs. 12–3 and 17–3). Multiple, irregular calcifications are characteristic of asbestos, and diaphragmatic calcification is pathognomonic of asbestos exposure. These pleural manifestations are benign clinically.

Asbestos is a major factor in the development of many malignancies, including carcinoma of the lung, malignant mesothelioma of the pleura and peritoneum and carcinoma of the stomach. Malignant mesothelioma of the pleura is an uncommon malignancy, and it rarely occurs without asbestos exposure. Radiographic findings include marked pleural thickening with or without associated nodules, and/or pleural effusion (Fig. 12–8). This form of malignancy is locally invasive and has an invariably fatal outcome. Benign mesothelioma is a local pleural mass that may be associated with pleural effusion but which is not related to asbestos exposure.

Twenty or more years after significant asbestos exposure a large percentage of those exposed develop lung cancer. Cigarette smoking in this population is synergistic, so that the combination of significant asbestos exposure and cigarette smoking eventually leads to lung cancer in alarming numbers of patients.

"BENIGN" PNEUMOCONIOSIS

MINERAL DUST

A large number of minerals cause pulmonary parenchymal abnormalities and occasionally may cause symptoms such as dyspnea and cough. Causes include iron, tungsten carbide, copper and aluminum. Chronic exposure does not usually produce disease as severe as silicosis or asbestosis, since the "benign" dusts stimulate little, if any, fibrotic reaction in the lung. Fine, interstitial nodules are the most common roentgenographic abnormalities seen (Fig. 17–1) and represent deposition of dust in the pulmonary interstitium that is usually far less symptomatic than the degree of roentgen abnormality would suggest. Since many of these minerals are mined from rock containing silica, it is important to remember that silicosis may occur in these same individuals.

ORGANIC DUST

A large number of organic particles, including some fungi, are capable of stimulating a hypersensitivity reaction (hypersensitivity pneumonitis, allergic alveolitis) in the lungs without causing an actual infection. Radiographic manifestations may be absent, but diffuse or patchy interstitial or alveolar patterns are common (Fig. 17–4). Repeated episodes can lead

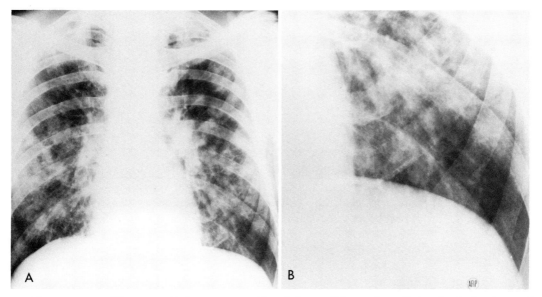

Figure 17–4. Hypersensitivity pneumonitis—"air conditioner lung." A mixed alveolar and interstitial infiltrate is evident on frontal view (A) and on closeup view of left lower lung field (B). Hila are enlarged bilaterally by lymph node enlargement, a finding in approximately 25 per cent of patients with this diagnosis. (AFIP negative #69–11208)

to pulmonary fibrosis with permanent respiratory impairment. Clinical history and laboratory studies confirm the diagnosis. One common example of this reaction is "farmer's lung," but the most common form in present clinical incidence is caused by organisms in air conditioning systems, heating systems and humidifiers.

ASPIRATION

GASTRIC CONTENTS

Unconscious or semi-conscious individuals may aspirate gastric contents. This is particularly common during anesthesia or after head trauma. Large amounts of acid material cause diffuse lung damage, which can be fatal immediately or after the development of secondary infection, adult respiratory distress syndrome or fibrosis. These patchy or diffuse areas of consolidation may resemble pulmonary edema (Fig. 17–5) or may be more irregular.

NASOPHARYNGEAL SECRETIONS

Unconscious or comatose patients aspirate pooled secretions from above. If significant quantities of virulent organisms are present, pneumonia and/or lung abscess may result. Pneumococcal pneumonia can occur by this mechanism. This is also the mechanism of lung abscess formation in patients with poor oral hygiene; anaerobic and microaerophilic organisms are aspirated, leading to a necrotizing pneumonia and lung abscess. Since gravity plays an important part in the distribution of these organisms within the lung, this form of lung abscess is typically seen in the posterior segment of the upper lobes or the superior segment of the lower lobes. A patient position other than supine can lead to an abscess in another segment. Foul breath or severe gum disease help make the initial diagnosis. Lung abscess is typically seen in alcoholics or after episodes of alcohol- or drug-induced unconsciousness.

INGESTED FOOD AND DRINK

Patients with neurologic disease, throat or esophageal abnormality due to congenital conditions, diverticula, neoplasm, trauma or surgery can aspirate during or after eating and drinking. This ingested material is typically less damaging to the pulmonary parenchyma than gastric contents of infected mouth and nasopharyngeal secretions. Patchy areas of consolidation without cavitation and frequently without symptoms are seen. Distribution again is related to the patient's position while aspirating. Since this is frequently erect, radiographic abnormalities are most common at the lung bases. Repeated episodes can lead to chronic pneumonia and/or fibrosis. If fatty material is aspirated (e.g., mineral oil) pulmonary tissue, reaction to the material may cause development of a chronic lipoid pneumonia, often a mass-like lesion easily mistaken for neoplasm.

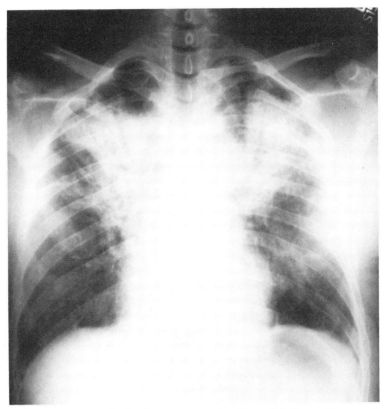

Figure 17–5. Aspiration pneumonia. Consolidation with prominent air bronchograms is present in both upper lung fields, especially the perihilar regions. The infiltrates are principally in the posterior segments of the upper lobes because the patient was apparently supine during aspiration following head trauma.

NEAR-DROWNING

Near-drowning is usually associated with inhalation of large quantities of fresh or salt water. These patients typically have the appearance of pulmonary edema or patchy consolidation (alveolar nodules) (Fig. 17–6). Secondary infection is common.

Laryngospasm is a common cause of death in drowning victims. Occasionally a nearly drowned patient will have a clear radiograph after the episode but hours to days later develop a pulmonary edema pattern presumably due to the adult respiratory distress syndrome (ARDS). Patients with typical near-drowning and pulmonary edema also can develop ARDS.

CONTRAST MATERIAL

Aspiration of contrast media used for evaluation of the esophagus and upper GI tract is common, since abnormalities of the swallowing mechanism or obstruction predisposes to aspiration. Barium sulfate is inert in the lungs but may remain for a long time if it reaches the peripheral airways. Hypertonic contrast media (e.g., Gastrografin and Hypaque) are irritating to the airways and lungs. Outpouring of fluid as a reaction to this material appears as pulmonary edema and can be fatal.

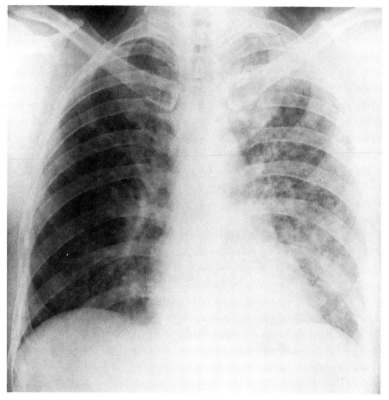

Figure 17–6. Near drowning. An alveolar nodular pattern is present in the left lung and, to a lesser extent, in the right lung. The patttern is not distinctive and could represent diffuse patchy pneumonia or pneumonitis. (AFIP negative #61–5948)

CHAPTER 18

CARDIOVASCULAR DISEASE

Special techniques to evaluate cardiovascular disease are beyond the scope of this book. Common plain film findings affecting the heart shadow, lungs and vessels (systemic and pulmonary) will be reviewed.

CONGENITAL VARIANTS

Situs inversus (complete side reversal, including stomach) and dextrocardia without situs inversus are easy to recognize if attention is paid to film labeling.

Although a right aortic arch often occurs with congenital cardiac anomalies, most right arches occur as isolated, insignificant findings (Fig. 18–1). Frequently dilatation of the origin of the left subclavian artery mimics a normal left arch in these patients. Clues to the correct diagnosis include impression of the right arch on the trachea and esophagus, a right-sided descending aorta, and a characteristic density behind the trachea and esophagus on the lateral film caused by the enlarged origin of the left subclavian artery.

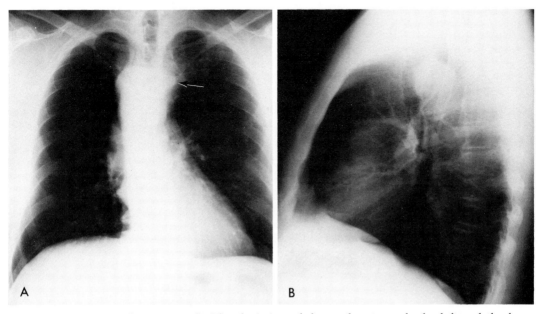

Figure 18–1. Right aortic arch. The deviation of the trachea towards the left and the large bulge in the right upper mediastinum are the obvious signs. Note the prominent left subclavian artery on the frontal view *(A)* (arrow). The marked anterior deviation of the trachea on the lateral view *(B)* is also obvious.

CARDIOMEGALY

Accurate determination of cardiomegaly is a difficult problem in chest film reading. Comparing maximum cardiac diameter to the thoracic diameter (CT ratio) is a frequently used guideline to determine an enlarged heart. Many use a CT ratio of 0.5 as the dividing point between normal and abnormal. Unfortunately the patient's body habitus and degree of inspiration greatly affect this measurement. It is only reliable as a way of following change when the inspiration taken is the same (see Fig. 18–15). Small amounts of change in the CT ratio as well as borderline values between 0.45 and 0.55 cannot be interpreted. Small but easily visible changes are often caused by comparison films exposed at different times in the cardiac cycle. Cardiac contour, clinical correlation, EKG and ultrasound findings are more useful. Other measurements of cardiac and vascular structures often have no clinical value because of normal variation and dependence on technical factors.

SPECIFIC CHAMBER ENLARGEMENT

Although evaluation of the cardiac chambers is often easily and more reliably done by clinical, EKG and ultrasound parameters, typical plain film findings are sometimes present. Enlargement of the ascending aorta is a good clue to left ventricular disease, and enlargement of the pulmonary arteries suggests right ventricular abnormality.

Characteristic patterns include:

Left Ventricle. Enlargement of the cardiac silhouette posteroinferiorly on the lateral view or a bulge of the lower left heart border on the frontal view (Figs. 18–2 and 18–3).

Right Ventricle. Enlargement of the cardiac silhouette anteriosuperiorly (retrosternally) on the lateral view.

Left Atrium. Impingement on the barium-filled esophagus on the lateral and RAO projections is the most sensitive evidence for left atrial enlargement (Fig. 18–4). Left atrial enlargement often causes a double density through the right side of the heart on the PA film, which, with increasing size, also displaces the left mainstem bronchus superiorly. On the PA film, convexity of the left heart border at the junction of the middle and upper thirds is often caused by an enlarged left atrial appendage. Enlargement of this structure is characteristic of rheumatic disease.

Right Atrium. Enlargement of this chamber is hard to separate by any plain film technique from right ventricular enlargement. Prominence of the superior right heart border on the PA film may be present.

AORTA AND BRACHIOCEPHALIC ARTERIES

Enlargement, tortuosity and calcification of the great thoracic arteries due to atherosclerosis occurs with increasing frequency after age 35. It is so common after 50 that it may be regarded as the rule rather than the exception. Aneurysms of these vessels are usually due to atherosclerosis. Syphilis, trauma, infection and predisposing congenital conditions are

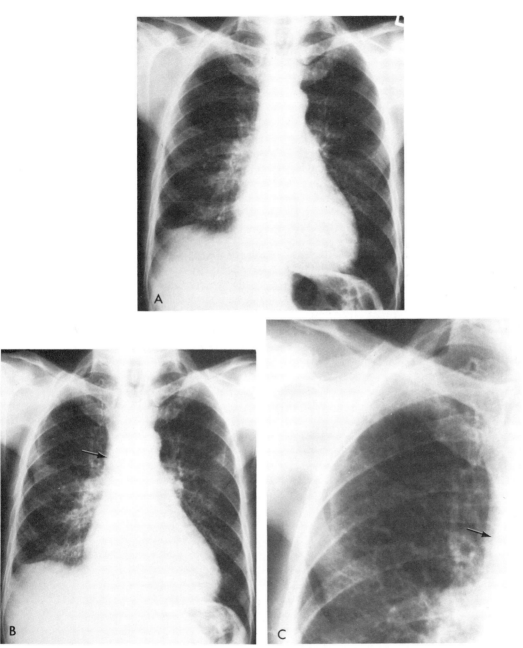

Figure 18–2.   Left ventricular enlargement with intravascular pulmonary congestion and dilated azygos vein. *A*, This view, obtained before this patient suffered a myocardial infarction, shows minimal dilatation of the heart and scarring of pleura near the diaphragm. The pulmonary vascularity is normal. *B* and *C*, Frontal view and closeup of right upper lung field following infarction show interval enlargement of the heart typical of left ventricular dilatation accompanied by dilated upper lung field vessels and dilation of the azygos vein (arrow). The superior mediastinum is also widened because of dilated systemic veins.

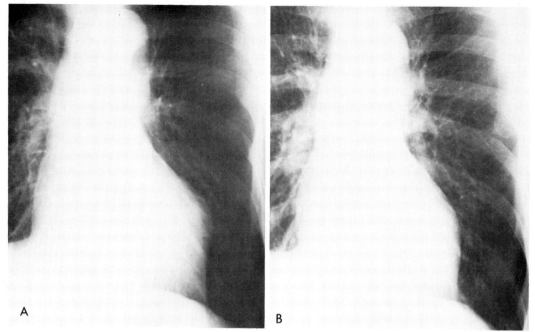

Figure 18–3. Left ventricular aneurysm. *A,* A distinct bulge is seen along the left heart border following a myocardial infarction with ventricular aneurysm formation. *B,* Previous film for comparison shows a normal left heart border.

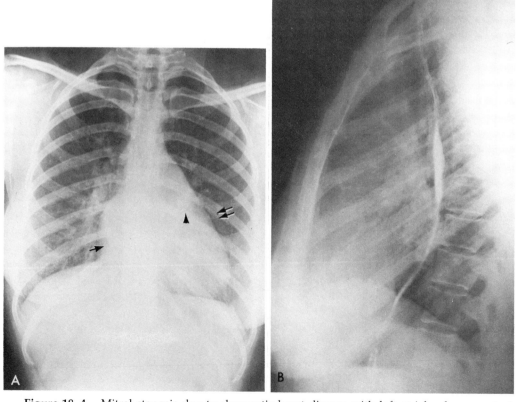

Figure 18–4. Mitral stenosis due to rheumatic heart disease with left atrial enlargement. *A,* Frontal view shows the left atrium bulging the right heart border (single arrow) and a convexity of the left heart border caused by enlargement of the left atrial appendage (double arrow). The left mainstem bronchus (arrowhead) is elevated. *B,* Lateral view with barium in the esophagus shows the left atrium indenting the anterior aspect of the lower esophagus. The esophagus returns to normal position before passing through the diaphragm.

other causes (Fig. 18–5). A calcified rim in a middle mediastinal mass strongly suggests aneurysm. Occasionally standard or computerized tomography is necessary to demonstrate this calcium, which is present in all but the most recently formed aneurysms.

Aortic dissection is usually caused by atherosclerosis or trauma or both and may dilate the aortic shadow dramatically (Fig. 18–6). Subtle dissection is often detectable by CT even when plain films show no changes, but aortography may be required for diagnosis.

Dilatation of the ascending aorta alone (Fig. 18–5) is commonly seen in aortitis, hypertension, syphilis and aortic valvular stenosis.

Coarctation of the aorta has several forms. The most common is called "adult" or "post-ductal" and consists of a local narrowing just distal to the orgin of the left subclavian artery. Since this is often a curable cause of hypertension, diagnosis is important. Radiographic signs (Figs. 18–7 and 18–8) include:

1. a break in the smooth contour of the proximal descending aorta, forming a notch. The coarcted segment itself may cause this notch, but most frequently the notch is at the site of the origin of the dilated left subclavian artery, which takes blood to collateral vessels, bypassing the coarctation.
2. a dilated left subclavian artery forming an extra superior mediastinal shadow above the aortic arch.
3. a prominent ascending aorta with a hypoplastic descending aorta.
4. rib notching, which characteristically occurs on the inferior rib margin in the middle third of the 3rd to 9th ribs bilaterally but may have an asymmetric distribution.
5. evidence of other dilated collateral vessels such as irregular retrosternal densities caused by the internal mammary arteries.

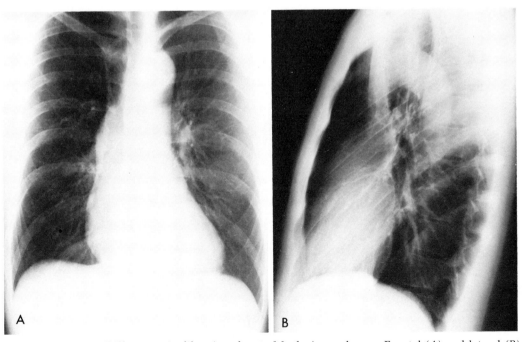

Figure 18–5. Diffuse aortic dilatation due to Marfan's syndrome. Frontal *(A)* and lateral *(B)* views show marked prominence of the ascending aorta and aortic arch without significant dilatation or tortuosity of the descending aorta. Such ascending aortic dilatation is also common in hypertension and post-stenotic dilatation from valvular aortic stenosis.

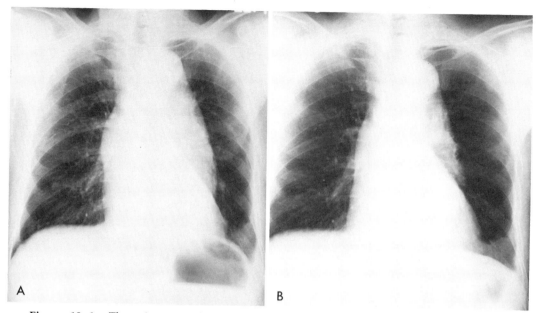

Figure 18–6. Thoracic aortic dissection. Frontal film (*A*) shows massive dilatation of the descending aorta not seen on a previous film (*B*) in this patient with severe chest pain. Without a comparison film, such dilatation of the descending aorta is far less diagnostic, as atherosclerotic dilatation alone may cause such an appearance.

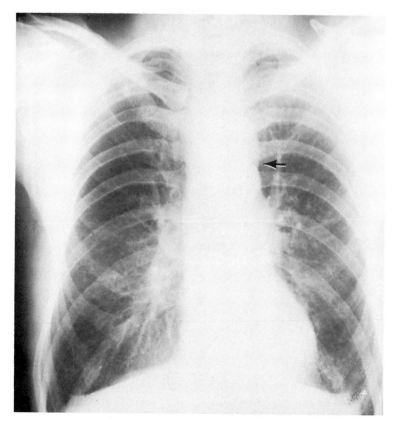

Figure 18–7. Pseudo-coarctation of the aorta. This example of an obvious break in the descending aortic shadow (arrow) is not a significant abnormality, as it represents a hemodynamically insignificant contour defect. The appearance in true coarctation of the aorta is often identical.

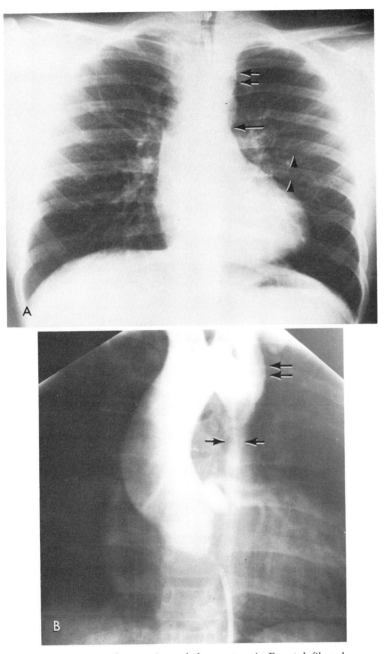

Figure 18–8. Coarctation of the aorta. *A,* Frontal film shows a far more subtle contour break (arrow) than in the previous case of pseudo-coarctation (Fig. 18–7). A dilated left subclavian artery (double arrow) is easily visible, the ascending aorta is prominent and subtle rib notching is seen (arrowheads). *B,* Contrast aortogram shows the marked narrowing in aortic contour (between arrows) and the dilated left subclavian artery (double arrow).

AZYGOS VEIN

The azygos vein travels cephalad, adjacent to the esophagus, and then arches anteriorly to join the superior vena cava. The anterior portion of this arch is often seen on end to the right of the trachea just superior to the origin of the right main bronchus (Fig. 18–2).

Enlargement (greater than 10 mm.) or increasing size of the azygos vein may be due to:

1. a normal variant or congenital anomaly.
2. congestive heart failure (especially right heart failure).
3. obstruction of the great veins with increased collateral flow through the azygous system.
4. portal hypertension.
5. constrictive pericarditis or pericardial tamponade.

CALCIFICATION

Since the cardiovascular structures are in constant movement, calcification, particularly if not extensive, is better seen fluoroscopically. Common calcifications include the following.

1. Plaque-like calcification in the walls of the aorta and brachiocephalic arteries is usually due to atherosclerosis.
2. Aortic and mitral valve calcification is almost invariably a sign of significant disease of these structures. Mitral calcification is usually due to rheumatic disease. Calcification of the aortic valve may be due to rheumatic disease or idiopathic calcific aortic stenosis. Often valvular calcification is seen only fluoroscopically.
3. Mitral annulus calcification, unlike valvular calcification, frequently is dense and flocculent and, thus, easily seen on standard films as a crescentic shadow in the middle of the heart (Fig. 18–9). This condition is idiopathic and usually of no clinical significance. It is common in elderly women.
4. Coronary artery calcification is very common (Fig. 18–10). It is a reliable indication of significant atherosclerosis in the involved vessel. Although tram-like calcifications in the coronary arteries are not uncommon on plain films, fluoroscopy is both more sensitive and more specific.
5. Pericardial calcification can be of any extent and can occur in any portion (Figs. 18–11 and 18–12). It is often sufficiently extensive and dense that it is seen on standard films. Previous pericarditis, often tuberculous, is the presumed etiology, but often no specific cause can be traced.
6. Myocardial aneurysms may calcify at the site of previous infarction. This is usually a small, linear calcification.

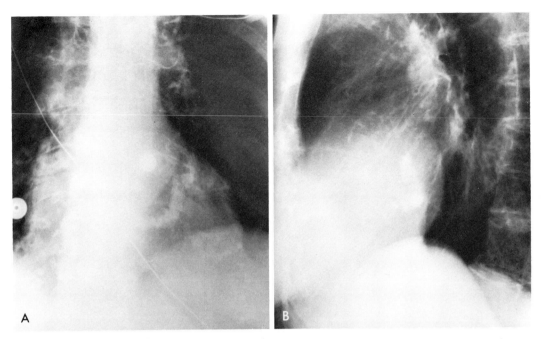

Figure 18–9. Mitral annulus calcification. Both frontal *(A)* and lateral *(B)* views show a prominent arch of calcification convex toward the diaphragm on the frontal view and toward the posterior heart border on the lateral view. Scattered calcifications are present in other vessels, bronchial walls and costochondral portions of anterior ribs in this elderly lady.

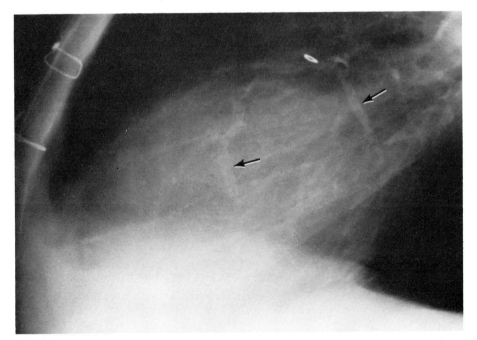

Figure 18–10. Coronary artery calcification. Unusually prominent coronary artery calcification is visible on this lateral view. A clip and sternal sutures are present because this patient has had a coronary artery bypass graft procedure.

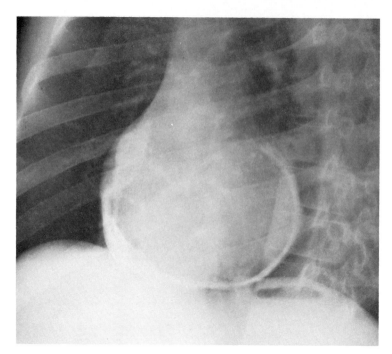

Figure 18–11. Tuberculous pericardial calcification. This oblique view shows the pericardium to be nearly completely calcified. Incidentally noted on this film is ossification of paraspinous ligaments secondary to ankylosing spondylitis.

Figure 18–12. Pericardial calcification, localized. This closeup view of the right heart border in an oblique projection reveals a thick area of calcified pericardium. This appearance is more typical than that in Figure 18–11.

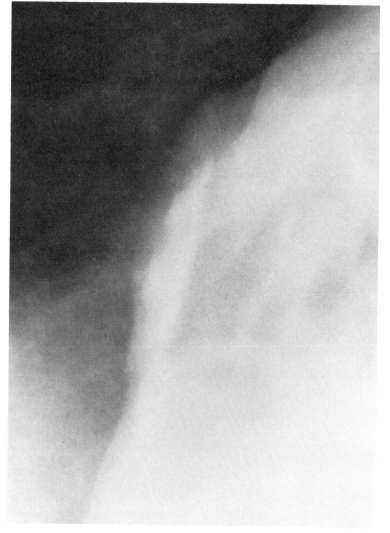

PERICARDIAL DISEASE

Pericardial effusion is much more accurately identified and quantitated by ultrasound. Occasionally, pericardial effusion is asymmetric or loculated, making diagnosis even more difficult without ultrasound. Plain film clues include a large amorphous cardiac silhouette, rapid change in size of the cardiac shadow and unexplained diffuse cardiomegaly, particularly if associated with pleural disease. In patients with abundant epicardial fat, a lucent stripe may be seen inside the apparent heart border. Lateral or oblique projections show this finding best. Fluoroscopy is much more sensitive in finding this "fat pad sign." Certain clinical conditions (e.g., uremia and systemic lupus erythematosus) should always suggest the possibility of pericardial effusion.

Partial absence of the pericardium (usually on the left side) may be congenital or due to surgery or to a penetrating wound. Rarely, herniation of all or part of the heart occurs through such a defect.

CONGESTIVE HEART FAILURE

Radiographic findings of congestive heart failure may precede clinical symptoms, especially in inactive individuals. Unfortunately these subtle changes are often difficult to be sure of, since technique, degree of inspiration, obesity and chronic lung disease all may cause confusing changes in the pulmonary vasculature and interstitial markings. Undercalling or overcalling radiographic congestive heart failure is frequent.

Right-sided heart failure may cause an increase in size of the azygos vein or superior vena cava, or both, and pleural effusion(s). Clues include enlargement of the right ventricle, enlargement of the pulmonary arteries (Fig. 18–13) and diffuse lung disease, especially COPD.

Most episodes of congestive heart failure are biventricular or left ventricular. At least three stages of left ventricular congestive failure are recognized. These stages always occur in the order given, but progression through the first two stages to pulmonary edema may be rapid. The greatest difficulty in radiologic diagnosis occurs in the more mild, early stages.

1. Intravascular Congestion. Normally, most of the blood flow through the pulmonary arteries and veins goes to the lower lung fields because of gravity. In early congestion, upper lobe vessels become dilated and more of them fill as the overall blood flow increases. In addition, some leakage of fluid into the interstitium of the lung occurs centrally (around the hilar structures) only. Thus, the radiologic findings in this stage (Fig. 18–14) are:

   a. upper lobe vessels equal to or greater than the diameter of lower lobe vessels.

   b. a haze or loss of definition of hilar and perihilar structures.

   c. minimal loss of definition of lower lung field vessels, especially behind the heart.

The lateral film may be especially helpful in detection of intravascular congestion. The areas superior to the heart and just above the arch of the aorta are useful places to compare the size of upper and lower lung field vessels and, especially, to compare vessel size with those on prior films. The inability to compare present films with previous films is the single greatest reason why intravascular congestion is often underdetected.

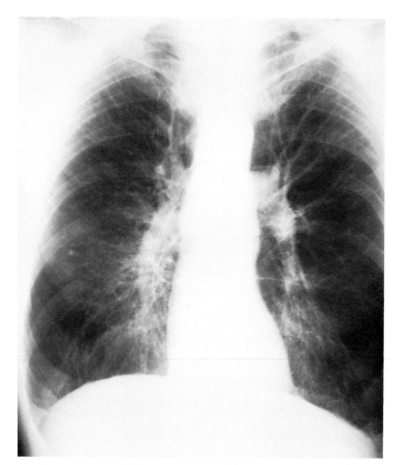

Figure 18–13. Pulmonary arterial hypertension secondary to chronic obstructive pulmonary disease. Frontal film shows upper lobe vessels that are larger than the vessels in the lower lung fields. It is clear that these vessels represent arteries because they can be followed centrally into very large pulmonary arteries on each side. It is important to distinguish this appearance from that of pulmonary venous hypertension (intravascular congestion), in which the prominent upper lobe vessels do not originate from large pulmonary arteries.

2. Interstitial Edema. In this stage, the intravascular pressure exceeds the ability of the vessels to contain the increased fluid load and leakage occurs into the pulmonary interstitium, especially thickening the paravascular and parabronchial portions of the interstitium. The radiographic signs (Figs. 18–14, 18–15 and 18–16) are:

    a. septal lines—Kerley B lines are especially prominent in interstitial edema, but Kerley A lines may also be seen.

    b. increasing blurring of lower lobe vessels and perihilar regions.

    c. irregular reticulations (Kerley C lines) and small indistinct nodules, especially in the lower lung fields. The small nodules are actually patchy regions of alveolar edema.

    d. thickening of fissures and pleural effusions often accompany interstitial edema but are actually manifestations of right-sided failure, as discussed above.

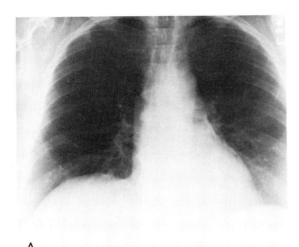

A

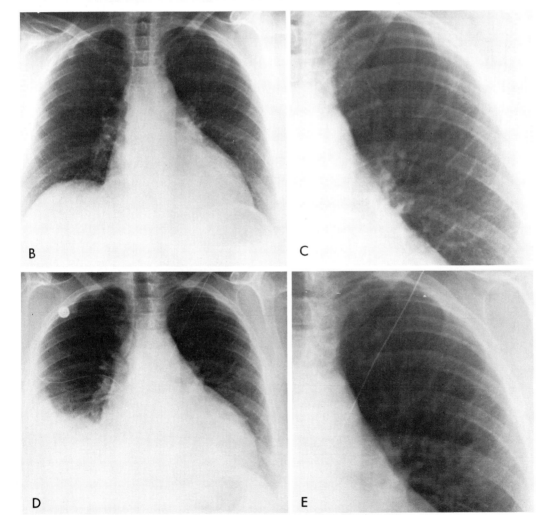

B

C

D

E

Figure 18–14. Congestive heart failure with intravascular congestion and interstitial edema. *A,* Frontal film made prior to present illness shows normal size heart and normal pulmonary vessels. Upper lobe vessels are nearly inapparent. *B,* With onset of symptoms, diffuse cardiomegaly is present, with dilated vessels and minimal haziness of the hila. The closeup view of the left upper lung field *(C)* shows the dilated upper lobe vessels not radiating from the left pulmonary artery. *D* and *E,* Two days later, increasing cardiomegaly is present, the azygos vein is dilated and there is now a large right pleural effusion. The upper lung field vessels *(E)* are dilated even more than previously *(B* and *C).* Lower lung field vessels are increasingly hazy, especially behind the heart, because of perivascular edema.

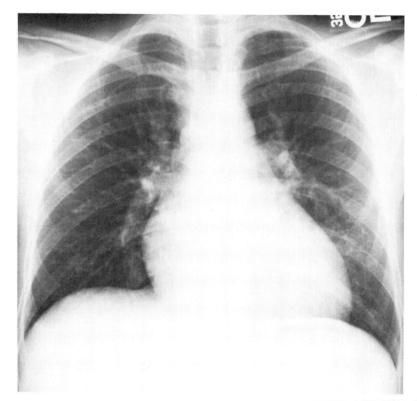

Figure 18–15. Congestive heart failure, interstitial edema. Frontal film shows diffuse reticulations, especially obvious in the left lower lung field. Upper lobe vessels are dilated, the azygos vein is enlarged and there is diffuse cardiomegaly. Lower lung field vessels are hazy and ill-defined.

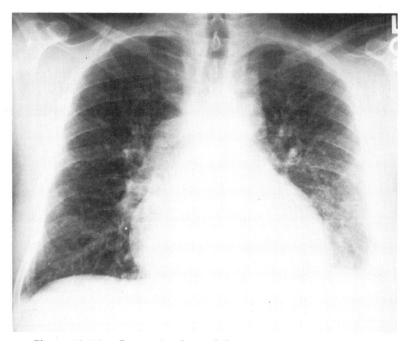

Figure 18–16. Congestive heart failure, severe interstitial edema. A marked reticular interstitial infiltrate is present, especially in the left lower lung field and, slightly less, in the right lower lung field. Upper lobe vessels remain dilated. Also noted is diffuse cardiomegaly, a dilated azygos vein, widening of the upper mediastinum due to venous distention and bilateral pleural effusions.

3. Alveolar (Pulmonary) Edema. In this most severe phase of congestion, the fluid pressure exceeds the intra-alveolar pressure of air and fluid flows into alveoli. The distribution is generally bibasilar or perihilar but may be diffuse in very severe cases. The radiographic signs (Fig. 18–17) are:

a. consolidative (alveolar) infiltration in perihilar regions ("bat wing" distribution) or bibasilar distribution. Air bronchograms may be prominent.

b. severe blurring of visible vessels in all portions of the lung fields, especially the lower lung fields.

c. Interstitial infiltration with septal lines and reticulations are usually present in those areas of lung in which consolidation is not present.

d. Thickened fissures and pleural effusions are common.

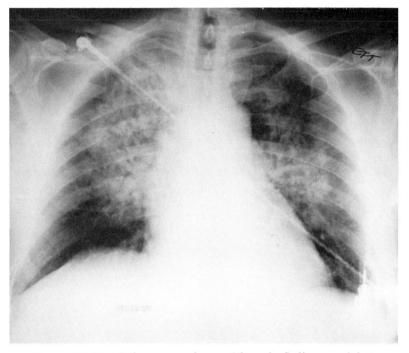

Figure 18–17. Pulmonary edema. Bilateral, fluffy consolidation is present in the perihilar regions with a typical "bat wing" distribution, sparing the periphery of both lung fields and the bases and apices. Prominent air bronchograms are present bilaterally, and there is some cardiomegaly.

CHAPTER 19

ICU AND IATROGENIC DISEASE

ICU

Intensive Care patients are critically ill, often requiring immediate decisions in life-threatening situations. The chest roentgenogram may show acute changes of atelectasis, aspiration, pneumonia, pulmonary embolism or edema in these patients, each requiring appropriate management.

The adult respiratory distress syndrome (ARDS) results from diffuse alveolar damage caused by a wide variety of insults, including shock, emboli, aspiration, infection and inhalation of toxic material. The damage to the alveoli causes edema, atelectasis and hyaline membrane formation. Radiographically, a pulmonary edema pattern with diffuse volume loss develops hours to days after the insult. A smooth ground-glass pattern (homogeneous, smooth opacity with scattered lucencies) is often seen and is more distinctive than nonspecific consolidation (Fig. 19–1). Clinical correlation and pulmonary wedge pressure may distinguish pulmonary edema due to congestive heart failure from ARDS, since the radiograph alone usually cannot. ARDS patients often require respiratory assistance with positive end expiratory pressure (PEEP). Variation in the level of PEEP causes a change in pulmonary volume and opacity, but this does not represent a change in disease severity. The radiograph can clear completely or may show scarring and atelectasis.

IATROGENIC DISEASE

The following are important complications of various procedures with radiographic correlates:

THORACENTESIS

Pneumothorax is common after this procedure. Rarely a hemothorax occurs.

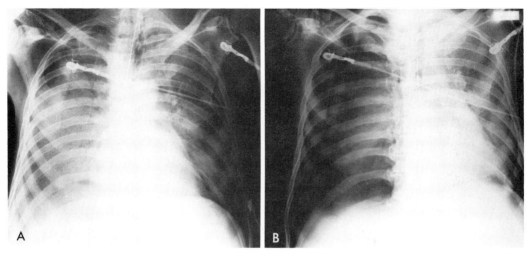

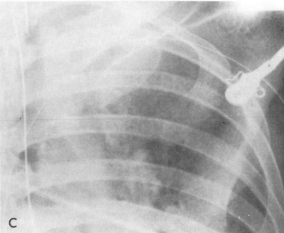

Figure 19–1. Adult respiratory distress syndrome. *A*, Frontal film of this patient with recent severe head trauma shows diffuse bilateral ground-glass infiltration with minimal volume loss. An NG tube, endotracheal tube and left CVP line are present. Note the diffuse homogeneity of the pulmonary infiltrate. *B*, Following initiation of PEEP, a large expansible right pneumothorax is seen. The pulmonary infiltrate remains unchanged. *C*, Closeup of left upper lung field shows lack of enlargement of upper lobe vessels and smoothness of infiltrate.

THORACOTOMY

1. Pneumothorax.
2. Hemorrhage into the pleural space, mediastinum or pericardial space.
3. Defects in the pericardium or diaphragm through which herniation may occur.
4. Leakage of the bronchial stump after pneumonectomy with aspiration of fluid from the post-pneumonectomy space into the remaining lung and subsequent infection of the post-pneumonectomy space.
5. Infections, including pneumonia, empyema, mediastinitis, and mediastinal abscess.
6. Atelectasis, most often of the left lower lobe.

TUBE AND CATHETER PLACEMENT

Correct positioning of the tip of a CVP line is in the superior vena cava or right atrium (Fig. 19–2).

Correct positioning of a Swan-Ganz catheter is in the left or right main pulmonary artery (Fig. 19–3).

The tip of a CSF shunt to the vascular system should be in the right atrium (Fig. 19–4).

Complications of placing these catheters may be present without a radiographically apparent catheter (some have been removed by the time the film is taken and others are radiolucent).

The complications include:

1. pneumothorax
2. pleural effusion
3. mediastinal widening due to fluid infusion
4. pulmonary infarct from a wedged Swan-Ganz catheter or embolism from clots originating on the catheter tip (Fig. 19–5)
5. superior vena caval obstruction from thrombosis
6. hemorrhage from a lacerated vessel or the heart

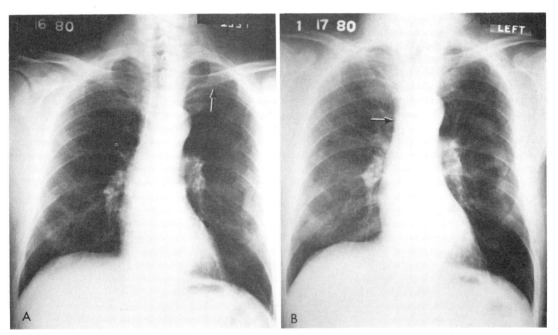

Figure 19–2. Central venous pressure (CVP) line. *A,* Initial frontal film shows a CVP line entering from the left arm through the left subclavian vein (arrow) that continues into the left jugular vein. *B,* One day later, a catheter has been repositioned so that its distal portion is now seen in the superior vena cava (arrow).

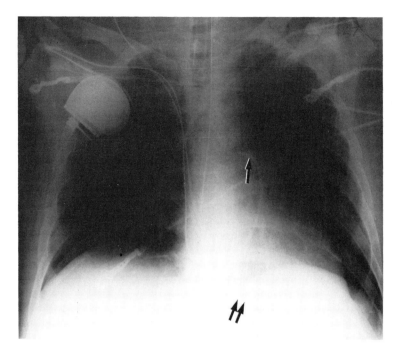

Figure 19–3. Swan-Ganz catheter. The catheter extends from the left arm through the venous system to the right atrium, right ventricle and pulmonary outflow tract with its tip in the main pulmonary artery (arrow). This patient, with a recent myocardial infarction, also has an endotracheal tube, a pacemaker on the right with its tip barely visible in the right ventricular apex (double arrow) and chest leads.

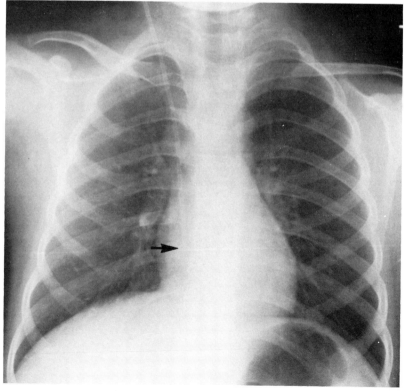

Figure 19–4. Cerebrospinal fluid (CSF) shunt. This catheter extends from the neck through the venous system with tip (arrow) in the right atrium.

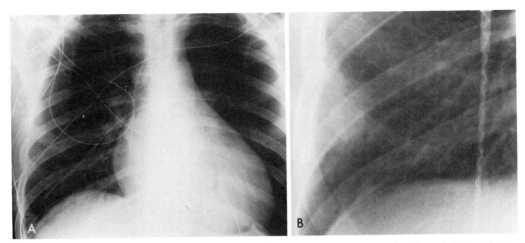

Figure 19–5. Distal Swan-Ganz catheter with subsequent pulmonary infarction. *A,* The catheter enters from the left arm and is seen through the heart with tip far distal in the right lower lobe pulmonary artery. *B,* Closeup view of right lower lung field made several days later shows a small peripheral consolidation with minimal pleural thickening and a convex border towards the hilum, typical of a small pulmonary infarct.

INTUBATION AND TRACHEOSTOMY

The trachea may be damaged by perforation or narrowing at the site of a stoma or where the tip of a tube or balloon abrades it (Fig. 19–6).

A malplaced endotracheal tube may damage the larynx or cause obstruction in either lung (usually the entire left lung or the right upper lobe), with resultant atelectasis and pneumonitis (Fig. 19–7).

Patients with diffuse lung disease on PEEP may develop interstitial emphysema as forced air dissects the alveolar lining (Fig. 19–8). This air can dissect back into the mediastinum and from there escape to subcutaneous tissues, the neck, the peritoneal space, the retroperitoneum and the pleural spaces. A resulting pneumothorax is life threatening in patients with severe respiratory compromise.

NASOGASTRIC TUBES AND ESOPHAGOSCOPY

Perforation of the esophagus causes mediastinal emphysema (Fig. 19–8), widening and often secondary infection. If the tip of a nasogastric tube is in the esophagus, it is not performing its function. Material infused through this tube may be aspirated by a nonalert patient.

Occasionally, an NG tube is found in the tracheobronchial tree (Fig. 19–9).

POST-RESUSCITATION

1. Fracture of ribs or sternum.
2. Pneumothorax.
3. Laceration of the heart or vessels.
4. Splenic rupture.

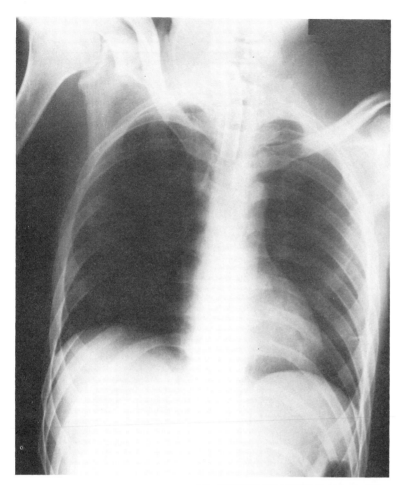

Figure 19–6. Tracheostomy tube and CSF shunt. The trach tube is in correct position in this patient. A ventriculo-peritoneal shunt is seen on the right traversing the mediastinum with tip not seen below the right hemidiaphragm.

Figure 19–7. Endotracheal tube in right mainstem bronchus. The tip of this endotracheal tube is approximately 2 cm. beyond the carina in the right mainstem bronchus. Massive consolidation of the left lung and infiltrate in the right lower lobe are seen with hyperaeration of the right upper lung field.

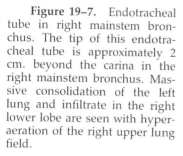

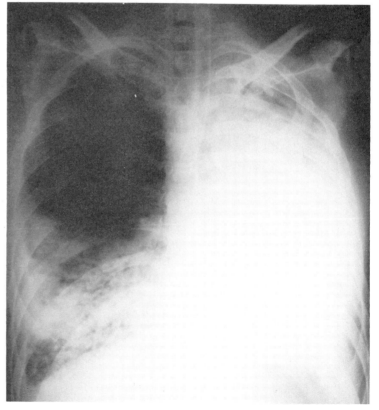

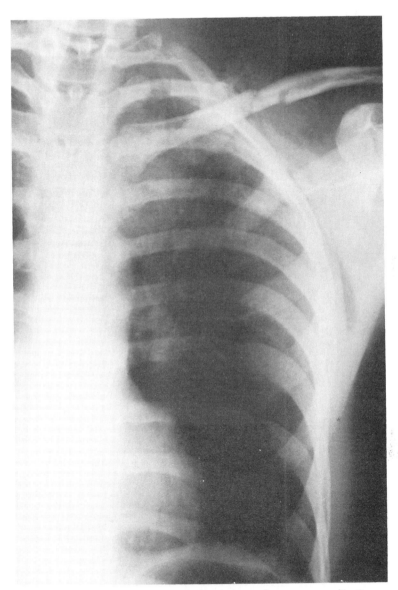

Figure 19–8. Interstitial emphysema and pneumomediastinum. This closeup view of the left upper lung field shows the appearance of air in the soft tissues of the shoulder, some of which is seen through the lung field and resembles an irregular infiltrate. The most medial irregular lucencies of air are probably also extending into the mediastinum.

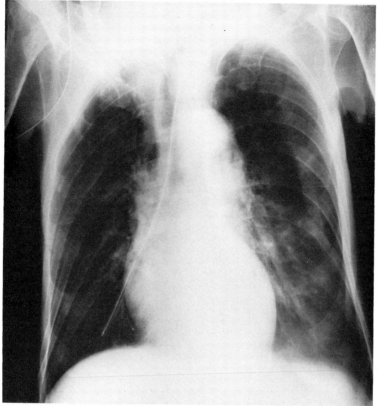

Figure 19–9. Nasogastric tube in right bronchus. The tip of this NG tube lies in a distal right lower lobe bronchus. The tube had been incorrectly introduced through the larynx and into the trachea.

TRANSBRONCHIAL AND PERCUTANEOUS NEEDLE BIOPSY

Pneumothorax is not uncommon after either of these procedures (Fig. 19–10). Pulmonary parenchymal bleeding can cause consolidation resembling pneumonia.

MEDIASTINOSCOPY

Hemorrhage may occur due to inadvertent biopsy of a vessel, causing a mediastinal mass or diffuse widening.

PACEMAKERS

The wires should be attached to the pacemaker, not broken or sharply angled.

The electrode of a transthoracic pacemaker is correctly implanted through the epicardium into the left ventricular myocardium.

A transvenous pacemaker catheter should be wedged in the apex of the right ventricle. Frontal and lateral projections are necessary to confirm this location (Figs. 19–11 and 19–12).

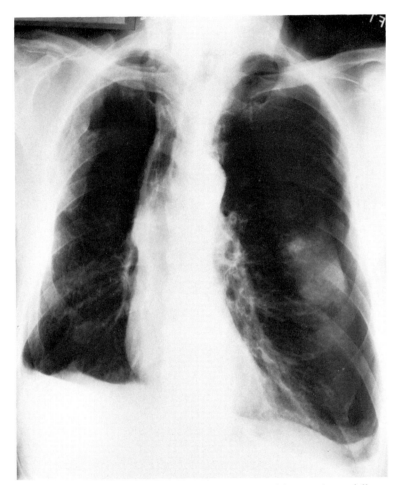

Figure 19–10. Pneumothorax and localized hemorrhage following transthoracic needle biopsy. A left pneumothorax with some expansion is visible. A consolidation in the periphery of the left midlung field is hemorrhage surrounding a pulmonary nodule (proved to be carcinoma) that was biopsied through the chest wall under fluoroscopic guidance.

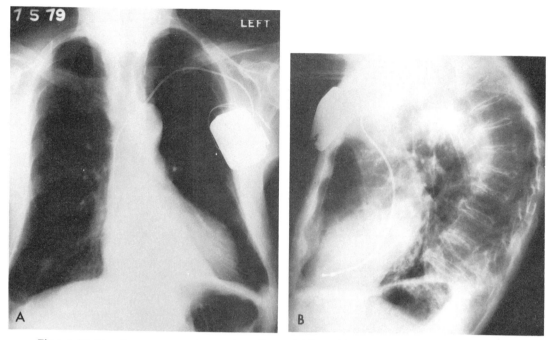

Figure 19–11. Transvenous pacemaker. Frontal *(A)* and lateral *(B)* views show a pacemaker on the left with leads traversing the venous system and ending in correct position at the right ventricular apex. Note especially the anterior position of the tip on the lateral view *(B)*.

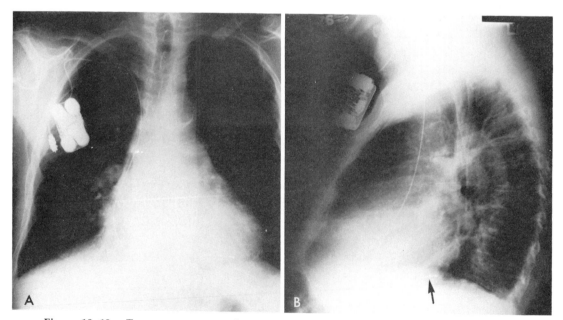

Figure 19–12. Transvenous pacemaker, incorrect tip position. On the frontal view *(A)*, the tip of the lead wire appears to extend farther to the left than is usual for the right ventricular apex. This impression is confirmed on the lateral view *(B)*, in which the tip (arrow) extends posteriorly and clearly lies within the left ventricle.

CHAPTER 20

SPECIAL PROCEDURES IN CHEST RADIOLOGY

Bronchography. Contrast material is used to coat the bronchi (Fig. 20–1). This allows the best radiographic picture of the large- and medium-sized airways. Current usage is limited. This technique remains the optimal way to document the diagnosis and extent of bronchiectasis before surgical resection of involved areas.

Bronchoscopy. Fiber optic bronchoscopy is often best done under fluoroscopic control to localize the position of the scope in relation to radiographically apparent abnormalities. Brushing and biopsy procedures through the scope are controlled by fluoroscopic monitoring.

Closed Cutting or Drill Biopsy. Fluoroscopic control allows correct positioning of the biopsy device. A good specimen is usually obtained, but significant morbidity and mortality due to damage of vessels and resultant hemorrhage are common (Fig. 19–10). This technique should be reserved for chest wall, pleural and pleural-based solid lesions to avoid serious complications.

Needle Aspiration. Fluoroscopic control is necessary to place the 18 to 23 gauge needle tip in the area of the abnormality. Diagnostic yield of this procedure is 75 to 90 per cent in malignancy but slightly less in inflammatory disease. This technique is safe for lesions anywhere in the thorax (less than 0.1 per cent mortality) when performed by an experienced individual. Mediastinal and hilar lesions may be safely sampled with this technique, since the aspirating needle rarely damages vital mediastinal structures even when it is misplaced. Following this procedure a chest tube for pneumothorax is required by 0.5 to 20 per cent of patients. A rare but serious complication of needle aspiration is severe hemorrhage, which very occasionally requires immediate surgery. The incidence of severe hemorrhage is greatest when cavitary lesions are biopsied.

Pulmonary Angiography. This is the definitive method of documenting pulmonary embolism and lesions of the pulmonary blood vessels (Fig. 20–2).

Thoracic Aortography. Congenital anomalies, aneurysms, dissection, laceration or occlusion of great arteries are evaluated by aortography.

Bronchial Arteriography. This procedure is currently used principally as part of an embolization procedure to control life-threatening hemoptysis.

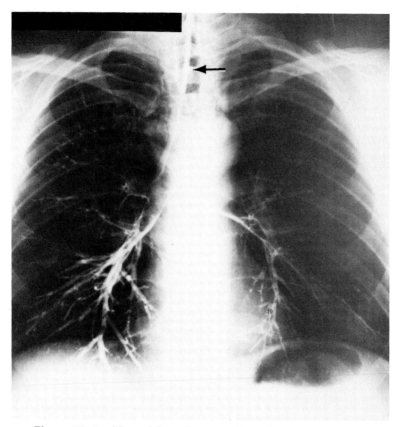

Figure 20–1. Normal bronchogram. Fat-soluble contrast material has been introduced into the tracheobronchial tree by a catheter, which is visible within the trachea (arrow). Contrast material lines the bronchi bilaterally and fills some of the distal bronchi, especially in the right lower lobe. Filling of each pulmonary segment is accomplished by turning the patient to use gravity.

Venography. Compression, obstruction and anomalies of the great veins can be evaluated by rapid arm injection of contrast or a catheter procedure.

Perfusion Radionuclide Lung (Q) Scan. A peripheral intravenous injection of radioactive particles which are trapped in the pulmonary capillaries allows the radionuclide demonstration of distribution of blood flow to the lungs (see Fig. 15–3).

Ventilation Radionuclide (V) Scan. An inhaled radioactive gas maps the distribution of inspired air. Followup scans show areas of air trapping (see Fig. 15–3).

Gallium Scan. This radioactive nuclide accumulates in many neoplasms and most inflammatory areas. It is a method of searching for site(s) of known or suspected disease.

Radionuclide Angiogram. A peripheral intravenous injection of tiny particles allows imaging of the heart and mediastinal great vessels. Recent improvements in technique and equipment allow this procedure to replace some standard angiograms.

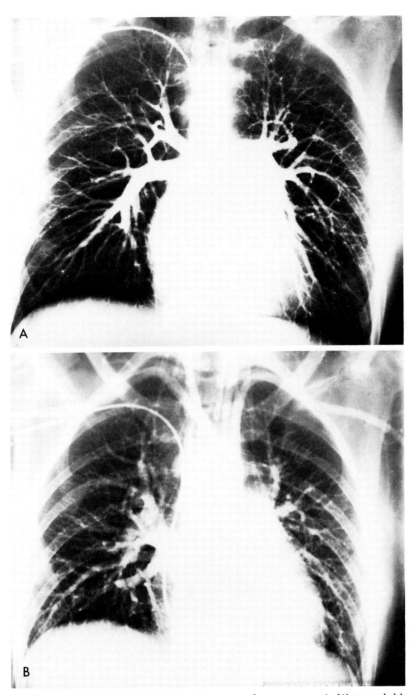

Figure 20–2. Pulmonary arteriogram and venogram. *A*, Water-soluble contrast material is filling the pulmonary arteries from a catheter entering via the right systemic veins, with catheter tip (not visible) in the main pulmonary artery. *B*, Later film from same injection shows the contrast now filling pulmonary veins, with some of the contrast already having passed through the left side of the heart into the systemic arteries. Note the inferior position of the pulmonary veins relative to the pulmonary arteries.

Subtraction Digital Angiography. Visualization of pulmonary, as well as systemic, vessels may be accomplished by using computer processing of an image produced by injection of contrast material into any peripheral vein. An image of exactly the same area, made prior to the injection, is subtracted from an image after injection, so that only the vessels are visualized. Because the resulting image is not as clear as with a selective arterial injection (Fig. 20–2), this technique has limited use within the chest but is sufficient for many abnormalities in the chest wall and other regions, such as the neck and limbs.

Computerized Tomography (CT). A computer-generated image of any plane through the body (axial, coronal, sagittal, oblique) is the result of a thin x-ray beam sent through the patient from multiple angles. A sensing system (e.g., a crystal) on the opposite side of the patient records the amount of x-rays passing through the patient at each angle and level. The computer registers all these inputs and creates an image on a television screen that can be photographed for a permanent record (see Fig. 13–5). This technique is of particular value in studying the mediastinum and chest wall.

Ultrasound. The use of high frequency sound waves is sometimes helpful for confirming and locating a pleural effusion. Cardiac ultrasound is widely applied in determining the nature of heart, pericardial and great vessel disease.

Nuclear Magnetic Resonance (NMR). The patient is placed in a magnetic field and the resonance of specific molecules (e.g., hydrogen) is selected out for recording. This allows determination of the concentration of that given substance in a particular area. There is no proven clinical use for this technique (as of 1982) but potentially it will allow assessment of physiologic conditions. Another advantage is that it does not require ionizing radiation to be passed through the patient.

GLOSSARY

air bronchogram — This is a sign first described by Felson. Normally the trachea, mainstem bronchi and occasionally the origins of the lobar bronchi are visible on chest radiographs as air-filled tubular structures. Visualization of more peripheral bronchi with air in them is usually not possible. Surrounding consolidation will sometimes allow these more peripheral bronchi to be seen as tubular or branching lucencies.

alveolar (consolidative) — An abnormal density is referred to by this term when its cause is the collapse or, more often, the filling of air spaces with abnormal material (usually "blood, pus, water, protein or cells"). Alveolar densities characteristically have irregular, hazy margins except where they are bounded by a pleural surface. Segmental distribution and air bronchograms are also characteristic of this pattern.

atelectasis — Collapse and volume loss are synonyms. Very small areas of atelectasis often produce a linear shadow, which is often, but not always, horizontal. This is referred to as plate-like, linear or subsegmental atelectasis. Lobar and total lung atelectasis also occur. These larger varieties of atelectasis are usually associated with increased density in the involved portion of lung so that there is, in fact, consolidation present as well. To diagnose atelectasis there must be specific evidence of volume loss such as displacement of a fissure, the mediastinum or a hilum. Elevation of the hemidiaphragm and decreased space between ribs can also be signs of atelectasis.

bleb — A small, thin-walled, air-containing structure. This term is frequently reserved for such small areas which are frequently intrapleural. This term may be used synonymously with "bulla" but often is reserved for smaller air spaces.

bulla — See "bleb" or "cavity." These abnormal air spaces may or may not be associated with diffuse pulmonary emphysema.

cavity — Another form of air space in the lung. This term is usually reserved for those which are the result of tissue necrosis, unlike bullae. Thickness and irregularity of the walls are often distinguishing features from bullae or blebs.

consolidation — Filling of pulmonary air spaces with some abnormal material may be referred to as either alveolar disease or consolidation.

density — A nonspecific term that can be used to describe any area of whiteness on the chest film. Normal structures such as the heart as well as abnormalities in the lungs may be called densities. This term is often used when the nature or cause of an abnormal shadow is not known. It is a useful term in that situation, since other terms (such as "mass" or "infiltrate") frequently imply more specific entities, which may or may not be present.

extra-pleural — Anything that is outside both the parietal and the visceral pleura but that impinges on the lungs may be described as extra-pleural. The heart is the most obvious example. Since normal or abnormal structures in this location are separated by two layers of pleura from the lung, the margins of these densities are characteristically sharp and smoothly tapering.

hilum (plural = hila) — The irregular medial shadow in each lung where the bronchi and pulmonary arteries enter. Other structures in these areas, particularly lymph nodes, are normally so small as to be inapparent. The normal hilar shadow is almost entirely composed of the central pulmonary arteries.

indeterminate or mixed lung disease—This category of diffuse lung disease is frequently used when the radiographic criteria used to designate a specific pattern (consolidative, interstitial, etc.) may not be present, or when there may be elements of several types of diffuse lung disease in the same patient.

infiltrate—A poorly defined abnormal pulmonary density or any such density sharply bounded by pleura and fissures. This is a confusing term, since it may be used by some to indicate any abnormal lung density and by others as a synonym for consolidation.

interstitial—The portion of the pulmonary parenchyma that consists of the actual lung tissue as opposed to the air spaces. Includes alveolar walls, septa, bronchovascular structures and pleura. Involvement of this tissue is a frequent form of diffuse lung disease.

kVp—Peak kilovoltage; the peak voltage across the x-ray tube. An increase in this factor allows increased tissue penetrance by higher energy x-rays.

lucency—An increase in blackness of an area on the radiograph. In the lung it may imply that air is being trapped, that lung tissue has been destroyed or that there is decreased blood supply. Artifacts, changes in position and soft tissue abnormalities can also cause areas of lucency.

mAs—Milliampere/seconds. This is the amount of current through the x-ray tube. The amount of current and the length of time during which the current flows control the quantity of x-rays generated. Increasing this factor (mAs) causes an increase in patient exposure to ionizing radiation and produces more x-rays to create an image on the film.

mass—A solid-appearing, reasonably well-defined soft tissue density usually larger than 3 or 4 cm. in diameter.

mediastinal—Referring to the structures or a lesion between the lungs. Unless the lungs are actually invaded by a mediastinal lesion, the lesion's x-ray shadow will be extra-pleural and, therefore, usually will have sharp demarcation from the lung.

miliary—A form of diffuse lung disease consisting of countless very tiny nodular densities.

nodule—A well-defined, more or less round density in the lung; smaller than a mass. No rigid size distinction between mass and nodule is possible.

opacity—Synonym for density.

pleural—Refers to an abnormality arising in the pleura or pleural space. Most commonly this is free or loculated fluid.

pneumothorax—Free air in the pleural space; may be modified by the following descriptive terms: hydro-, pyo-, hemo-, chylo-, tension.

pulmonary edema—As a radiographic term, diffuse, bilateral consolidation by fluid is called pulmonary edema. Other materials can fill air spaces bilaterally and give the same radiographic patterns.

reticular—A fine branching pattern with lines radiating in all directions; one of the signs of the interstitial pattern.

segmental—Limited to specific bronchopulmonary segments or lobes. Segmental distribution of disease usually indicates bronchial or vascular involvement and is most common in consolidation.

septal (or Kerley) lines—Thickening of interlobular septa for any reason may allow them to be seen as narrow straight shadows especially at the periphery of bases (Kerley "B" lines); another form of interstitial abnormality.

silhouette sign (Felson)—Normally an interface is seen between areas of different density as between shadows of the heart and lung. Loss of air on the pulmonary side usually because of consolidation may cause obliteration or "silhouetting" of this normal interface. This sign is useful in localizing an abnormality or confirming the presence of abnormality. Occasionally the silhouette sign will be the only definite indication of consolidation next to the heart or diaphragm.

BIBLIOGRAPHY

INTRODUCTORY MATERIAL

1. Felson, B.: *Chest Roentgenology*. Philadelphia, W. B. Saunders Co., 1973.
2. Squire, L. F.: *Fundamentals of Roentgenology*. Rev. ed. Cambridge, Harvard University Press, 1975.
3. Thompson, T. T.: *Primer of Clinical Radiology*. Boston, Little, Brown & Co., 1980.

REFERENCE

1. Fraser, R. G., and Paré, J. A. P.: *Diagnosis of Diseases of the Chest*. 2nd edition in 4 vols. Philadelphia, W. B. Saunders Co., 1977–79.

DIFFERENTIAL DIAGNOSIS

1. Lillington, G. A., and Jamplis, R. W.: *A Diagnostic Approach to Chest Diseases*. 2nd edition. Baltimore, Williams and Wilkins, 1977.
2. Reed, J. C.: *Chest Radiology: Patterns and Differential Diagnoses*. Chicago, Year Book Medical Pubs., 1981.

SPECIAL PROCEDURES

1. Sagel, S. S.: *Special Procedures in Chest Radiology*. (SMCR, vol. 8). Philadelphia, W. B. Saunders Co., 1976.
2. Kreel, L.: Computed tomography of the lung and pleura. *Seminars in Roentgenology* 13:213, 1978.
3. Heitzman, E. R., Goldwin, R. L., and Proto, A. V.: Radiological analysis of the mediastinum utilizing computed tomography. *Seminars in Roentgenology* 13:277, 1978.

INDEX

Page numbers in italics indicate illustrations; page numbers followed by t indicate tables.